MEDICAID
IN THE
REAGAN
ERA

MEDICAID IN THE REAGAN ERA Federal Policy and State Choices

Randall R. Bovbjerg
John Holahan

An Urban Institute Paperback

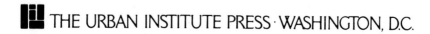 THE URBAN INSTITUTE PRESS · WASHINGTON, D.C.

THE URBAN INSTITUTE is a nonprofit policy research and educational organization established in Washington, D.C. in 1968. Its staff investigates the social and economic problems confronting the nation and government policies and programs designed to alleviate such problems. The Institute disseminates significant findings of its research through the publications program of its Press. The Institute has two goals for work in each of its research areas: to help shape thinking about societal problems and efforts to solve them, and to improve government decisions and performance by providing better information and analytic tools.

Through work that ranges from broad conceptual studies to administrative and technical assistance, Institute researchers contribute to the stock of knowledge available to public officials and to private individuals and groups concerned with formulating and implementing more efficient and effective government policy.

Conclusions or opinions expressed in Institute publications are those of the authors and do not necessarily reflect the views of other staff members, officers or trustees of the Institute, or of any organizations which provide financial support to the Institute.

CONTENTS

TABLES

FOREWORD

This report on recent Medicaid developments is a product of The Urban Institute's three-year examination of "Changing Domestic Priorities" under the Reagan administration. Funded by a consortium of foundations and corporations, this project is analyzing changes in federal economic and social policy and how they affect people, places, and institutions.

The administration's major goals for Medicaid have been to cut federal spending and transfer much more responsibility for program design and financing of cost increases to the states. Accordingly, the president proposed placing a 5 percent "cap" on federal spending growth, as against a projected 15-20 percent, and reducing federal requirements significantly to allow states to redesign the scope and content of their support for indigents' medical care. Medicaid would have operated more like a fixed federal block grant to states rather than as a jointly underwritten entitlement to specified services.

Congress rejected such a broad devolution of previous federal commitments. The Omnibus Budget Reconciliation Act of 1981 retained a larger federal role and financial responsibility along with less thoroughgoing state discretion than the president had sought. Although Congress thus maintained the basic nature of the federal-state Medicaid partnership, it nonetheless did further encourage states to economize by reducing federal matching assistance by 3 percent. It also significantly increased state flexibility to make economizing changes, especially in hospital payment methods.

Medicaid has grown to be the largest single state program in many states, and controlling its spending has long been a high state priority. States' own fiscal pressures exceed those newly imposed by Congress, and Medicaid programs have already been quite inventive in seeking to restrain Medicaid costs, with the least harmful restrictions on eligibility and services. Thus, Medicaid economizing under the Reagan administration represents as much continuity as change.

Bovbjerg and Holahan analyze states' economizing choices before and after the 1981 federal changes. They provide a useful anatomy of the program and a natural history of its endemic cost problems in an era of rapid medical price inflation. This study explains how state choices (within federal guidelines) have structured each state's program and determined its spending and, conversely, how the various options for constraining spending would redesign the program.

Special attention is given to two dilemmas facing economizers: (1) Cutting spending reduces access to care for program beneficiaries who must compete with better insured private and Medicare patients; and (2) Medicaid cuts also reduce federal support for indigent care, much of which may instead wind up being provided entirely at state and local expense, in public hospitals, or through general assistance medical programs. The authors give a practical perspective to their analysis by reporting in some detail on recent developments in ten states. Changes in eligibility, service coverage, utilization controls, provider payment methods, and other measures are all considered.

More Medicaid changes are under consideration in Washington and in state capitols. We hope this timely Medicaid analysis, as well as the other research to be published in this series, will promote more informed public policy and better decision making during an era of fundamental reconsideration of national goals.

John L. Palmer
Isabel V. Sawhill
General Editors
Changing Domestic Priorities Series

ACKNOWLEDGMENTS

We would like to thank our Urban Institute colleagues, especially William Scanlon and Judith Feder, for their support and constructive criticism. Among the many helpful outside contributors to our understanding of Medicaid developments, Richard Curtis and Lawrence Bartlett of the National Governors Association deserve special mention. We only wish space permitted us to acknowledge our debts to the many state Medicaid officials who have been so generous with their time and data and without whom this type of work would be impossible. Priscilla Taylor very competently edited our manuscript, which was typed and retyped by Johnetta Ward and Lanette Simmons.

This report was written with support from a consortium of private foundations and corporations under the auspices of The Urban Institute's Changing Domestic Priorities project. It draws upon numerous past Health Policy Center projects, as well; The Fiscal Limitations study under contract no. HEW-100-79-0174 from the U.S. Department of Health and Human Services provided the most direct input. The authors' opinions and any factual errors should not, of course, be construed to be those of the Institute or its sponsors.

Randall R. Bovbjerg
John Holahan

ABOUT THE AUTHORS

RANDALL R. BOVBJERG is a lawyer and a senior research associate in the Institute's Health Policy Center. He has recently studied how state and local health policy has been affected by fiscal limitations on state revenues or expenditures and by federal changes in Medicaid and other grant programs. He has also investigated how litigation has helped shape state hospital rate setting and health planning efforts. Before joining The Urban Institute he was state insurance regulator in Massachusetts. Mr. Bovbjerg's publications include articles on competition and regulation for the *Vanderbilt Law Review* and on competition and Medicare's End Stage Renal disease program for *Seminars in Nephrology*.

JOHN F. HOLAHAN is director of the Health Policy Center at The Urban Institute. He has recently completed a major study of physician reimbursement policy in the Medicare and Medicaid programs and has coordinated a project that examined a wide variety of problems in implementing national health insurance. He is the author of *Financing Health Care for the Poor*, coeditor of *National Health Insurance: Conflicting Goals and Policy Choices*, and coauthor of *Insuring the Nation's Health: Market Competition, Catastrophic and Comprehensive Approaches*. He is currently conducting a study of the effects of alternative reimbursement systems on nursing home cost inflation.

INTRODUCTION AND SUMMARY

This report assesses the Reagan administration's Medicaid policies, the changes Congress made in the law in 1981, and the states' responses.[1] The report focuses on causes of spending and on cost containment. The first chapter briefly describes the historical structure of the Medicaid program and the recent modifications of it. The second chapter analyzes the history of the program's cost problems; the states' cost-containment efforts; and the legal, political, and (ironically) fiscal constraints on effective action. The third chapter considers in some detail the cost-containment choices that have been and are now available to states and the ways they are being used. Chapter four provides the conclusions of this study.

Medicaid is a joint federal-state (and, occasionally, local) medical assistance program that pays for certain medical services provided to certain low-income individuals and families. How best to control Medicaid spending has become an increasingly important public policy issue for both state and federal governments since the mid-1970s. This report primarily discusses these past half dozen years through federal fiscal year (FY) 1982. It draws upon official program statistics (which are, unfortunately, available only through calendar 1979), considerable past Urban Institute research, other secondary sources, and many interviews with knowledgeable Medicaid administrators and analysts. Interviews were especially useful for insights about major changes since the 1981 Omnibus Budget Reconciliation Act.[2] We do not address FY 1983 proposals in any detail.

Recent efforts to economize need to be examined against the backdrop of earlier program developments, because the recent efforts really represent an intensification of earlier cost-containment efforts

by the states—which have in fact continued almost independent of
the stimuli of the 1981 act. Indeed, many of the provisions of the
1981 act drew upon earlier experience in path-breaking states. Since
Medicaid is an entitlement program, new fiscal controls cannot be
directly applied through budget limits and administrative directives
but must work indirectly by altering a state's program design. Thus
to understand the newly implemented changes it is important to
understand previous federal and state choices about the original
scope and structure of the program(s) as well as previous efforts to
economize.

Particular federal rules are only one determinant of how much
a state spends on Medicaid and of where and how a state will cut
expenditures if it must. The poor and chronically ill everywhere
need some medical care but are unable to pay for it. Almost everywhere some government support, whether state or local, is thought
desirable, but different jurisdictions provide varying degrees of assistance. Given such state and local spending, states find open-ended
federal Medicaid matching grants a very attractive way to help
finance this burden for at least some of their disadvantaged population. Conversely, many Medicaid cuts would simply leave states

and localities to bear the burden of financing care without federal
aid. Thus, states typically want to maintain a basic structure of
Medicaid despite the 1981 act's marginal reductions in the federal
percentage share and its considerable increases in state discretion
to cut Medicaid programs.

There is, however, great and increasing interest among the states
in improving program efficiency and in making marginal program
adjustments to conserve ever-more-limited state tax dollars. Very
recently, some states have made or are contemplating quite major
changes. Our review of these developments leads us to these conclusions:

1. Recent increases (since 1973) in Medicaid expenditures are
attributable to a general increase in the prices for all health care,
and, to a lesser extent, expansion of service coverage that has been
encouraged by federal matching funds.

2. Although the 1981 act was an important factor in bringing
about Medicaid program contractions in FY 1982, general economic
conditions and the fiscal conditions of particular states were more
important influences.

3. The change in Medicaid's hospital payment policy was the most important part of the 1981 act. Now freed from the necessity to base payments on what each hospital spends, several states are changing payment methods to control growth in rates. Many states also are limiting covered hospital days (always permissible) more tightly than ever before. As yet, no states have implemented new systems to "lock out" from Medicaid payment hospitals that are deemed too expensive.

4. There have been reductions in eligibility for Aid to Families with Dependent Children (AFDC) and thus in Medicaid costs both from cuts required in the 1981 act and from longer-term state freezes in welfare payment standards. In general, states have not made drastic cuts in Medicaid eligibility because the result would be a shift of costs to local government or private payers, particularly for care in public hospitals and for nursing homes.

5. Nursing home rates have not recently been sharply curtailed in most states. (Although federal requirements for nursing homes payment were loosened by the 1980 Omnibus Reconciliation Act, rather than the 1981 act, the changes were not implemented until 1981.) The relative stability of nursing home rates largely reflects the fact that most states had already established reasonable control over rate increases in recent years, particularly when compared with rates for hospitals. Hospital cost control dominates 1981-1982 developments.

6. Physician fees for services to Medicaid patients continue to be controlled in most states at levels that are low by standards of private or Medicare fees. Low physician participation continues to be a problem, hurting beneficiaries' access to doctors and sometimes actually increasing spending when more expensive hospital-based care is substituted.

7. Many states have applied or are planning to apply for several waivers to alter the structure of their Medicaid programs in major ways (e.g., under the new freedom of choice, case management, and community-care waiver provisions). But no significant savings are expected, particularly in the short run. In the long run, the prospect for savings is mixed; community care in particular may increase spending.

8. There have been few cutbacks in Medicaid coverage of the major optional services, such as intermediate care facilities, but limitations are commonly placed on smaller optional benefits, particularly prescription drugs.

As this listing shows, states have been quite inventive in administering and even redesigning their Medicaid programs to slow growth in spending. Their record of innovation, even under federal regulation, compares very favorably with Medicare and even with private insurance. Indeed, the states "earned" the new discretion conferred on them by the 1981 act in the sense that most of the 1981 provisions were modeled upon prior efforts by states to economize.

Most states are now constraining the scope of their programs more than ever before, but there are clear limits on their willingness to reduce their programs. Cost containment is not the overriding goal; costs, federal assistance, and medical care for the poor and chronically ill must all be reconciled. This reconciliation is not a simple problem for which standard solutions exist, and states have taken numerous different approaches depending on their individual circumstances and preferences. Despite the administration's efforts to "cap" the Medicaid program and make it more like a closed-end block grant, Congress has maintained the basic character of the program as open-ended assistance to fund entitlements to care. Accordingly, states have continued to avail themselves of the federal matching grants rather than seek drastic program curtailments that would hurt beneficiaries and providers as well as cost the states federal funds.

CHAPTER 1

AN OVERVIEW OF PRE-1981 DEVELOPMENTS AND 1981 CHANGES IN THE LAW

Understanding Medicaid policy choices in the wake of President Reagan's proposals to realign federal and state roles calls for some background. This chapter briefly reviews the basic Medicaid program structure and the history of spending increases as a backdrop to the 1981 federal changes proposed by the administration and to the changes enacted by Congress. To encourage states to economize further, Congress increased both the fiscal pressures on the states and their discretion to implement many cost-containment strategies previously impeded by federal policy. Later chapters cover the causes of spending rises in the past and state responses in the past, present, and future. In large measure the 1981 federal statute to cost increases—the Omnibus Budget Reconciliation Act—attempts to give all states the benefit of some states' pioneering efforts to promote program efficiency and to conserve tax dollars.

Structure of Medicaid

As has already been pointed out, Medicaid is a joint federal-state (and, occasionally, local) medical assistance program that pays for certain medical services provided to certain low-income individuals and families. Although many poor people are not covered, Medicaid is the principal payer for health care for the poor and significantly affects the residual financial burden borne by state and local welfare systems and by public hospitals.

The federal statute establishing the program, Title XIX of the Social Security Act, makes available federal matching grants to states choosing to establish and administer a program. With the recent addition of Arizona, all states now participate.[1] Despite the changes made by the 1981 act (discussed in detail later), the basic structure of Medicaid still follows its traditional pattern. Persons eligible for the AFDC and Supplemental Security Income (SSI) cash-assistance programs are automatically eligible for Medicaid; in addition states can choose to cover several other categories of individuals, most notably the "medically needy" (people whose large medical spending lowers them to welfare levels). States are required to provide hospital inpatient care, physician services, skilled nursing facility care, laboratory and x-ray services, home health services, and hospital outpatient care; if they so choose, states can provide 32 other services, including care in intermediate care facilities and mental hospitals, prescription drugs, and dental services.

Medicaid is a vendor-payment program operated as "third-party" coverage. That is, state programs pay bills for services decided upon by the two principals in the transaction, patients and providers. Payment is made directly to providers (typically, nursing homes, hospitals, and physicians) rather than to beneficiaries. Once eligible, a beneficiary is entitled to receive any covered service from any qualified provider of medical care.[2] (States now can limit this "free choice of provider" for beneficiaries, as will be discussed later.) Because of the open-ended "entitlement" nature of the program, states can assert fiscal control only by changing their programs—eligibility standards, services covered, and the like—and not by implementing direct controls on number of beneficiaries, total spending, and so on.

The federal government, which matches state expenditures for care on a percentage-of-payment basis, thus also faces open-ended liabilities.[3] The federal matching percentage is inversely related to a state's per capita income relative to the national average. Thus, larger contributions are made on behalf of poorer states. The maximum federal share in 1980 was 77.55 percent; seventeen states received the minimum 50 percent federal match. (The 1981 act slightly lowered the matching amounts payable, as is explained later.)

As of FY 1979 only nine states required localities to contribute to Medicaid programs, and the local share is very small everywhere but New York. Sometimes local authorities are responsible for a portion of program administration, notably determination of eligibility.

Although federal statute and regulations established the basic structure of Medicaid programs, states have long had considerable autonomy to set the basic scope of their programs—as well as to choose specific cost-controlling strategies. (State discretion was increased in 1981.) Nonetheless, whether a particular state action is consistent with federal law is ultimately determined by federal administrative review or the courts.

State Medicaid Spending

By any measure, Medicaid is the dominant factor in states' health budgeting. The program is huge, with some $37.2 billion nationwide estimated for FY 1983, of which the states' share is expected to be some $17.1 billion.[4] Medicaid now accounts for about a third of state and local health care expenditures and is often the largest program in a state's budget.[5]

Medicaid spending has increased rapidly since the program's inception. Nationally, Medicaid payments to medical providers[6] rose at an annual rate of 15.5 percent from FY 1973 to 1979 (the last year with complete data). Table 1 shows 1973 and 1979 expenditures as well as annual rates of increase for all states. The state with the lowest annual rate of increase was Maryland, at 7.2 percent. Alaska had the highest annual rate of 41.8 percent. Twenty states had rates of increase that exceeded 20 percent. Since FY 1979, higher spending trends have not abated, but some of the reasons behind the growth in expenditures have changed, as is discussed in the next chapter.

Since about 1975, moreover, longer-term pressures have been building on Medicaid budgets, as well as on the state budgets of which they have become so large a part. State revenues as a proportion of the gross national product have declined since the mid-1970s,[7] and Medicaid rates of increase in spending have almost everywhere outpaced growth in other state spending or in revenues—often by one-third to one-half more. (There are, of course, exceptions, notably Maryland and New York, where programs in the late 1970s succeeded in containing costs considerably.

Although pre-1973 rates of growth in Medicaid spending were even larger, as programs built up from scratch during the late 1960s, more recent growth has caused more political problems. (See table 2 in chapter 2.) Recent increases have been larger in absolute terms because they came on top of a much larger base of spending. Moreover, only some of the recent increase has gone to buy new benefits or to cover new people; most stems from extraordinary rates of cost increase, as is explained later. Finally, political attitudes toward

TABLE 1

GROWTH RATES OF MEDICAID EXPENDITURES BY STATE,
FISCAL YEARS 1973 AND 1979

State	FY 1973 (In $ millions)	FY 1979 (In $ millions)	Average Annual Compound Percentage Increase
Alabama	79.57	239.57	20.17
Alaska	3.28	26.66	41.80
Arkansas	45.61	192.23	27.09
California	1,087.86	2,557.91	15.31
Colorado	74.02	162.86	14.04
Connecticut	118.75	296.25	16.46
Delaware	11.11	38.41	22.97
District of Columbia	63.05	139.42	14.14
Florida	97.80	341.58	23.18
Georgia	177.49	382.81	13.67
Hawaii	30.56	86.30	18.89
Idaho	16.07	44.87	18.66
Illinois	480.47	991.83	12.84
Indiana	125.57	314.60	16.54
Iowa	36.96	208.35	33.34
Kansas	73.50	164.38	14.36
Kentucky	73.73	248.76	22.47
Louisiana	80.85	342.34	27.19
Maine	43.30	114.08	17.52
Maryland	171.05	258.81	7.15
Massachusetts	380.37	901.84	15.48
Michigan	426.81	1,036.40	15.93
Minnesota	182.10	474.42	17.30
Mississippi	55.59	148.60	17.81
Missouri	68.15	238.63	23.23
Montana	16.98	52.97	20.88
Nebraska	41.03	94.34	14.89
Nevada	11.67	32.15	18.40
New Hampshire	11.45	60.06	31.82
New Jersey	248.99	659.45	17.63
New Mexico	20.03	58.43	19.53
New York	2,260.96	3,860.59	9.33
North Carolina	107.83	336.70	20.90
North Dakota	15.10	41.79	18.49
Ohio	221.26	669.87	20.27
Oklahoma	114.83	251.49	13.96
Oregon	31.70	162.05	31.24
Pennsylvania	405.94	1,187.82	19.60
Rhode Island	57.59	139.91	15.95

TABLE 1 (continued)

State	FY 1973 (In $ millions)	FY 1979 (In $ millions)	Average Annual Compound Percentage Increase
South Carolina	45.05	191.41	27.27
South Dakota	14.74	48.97	22.15
Tennessee	68.90	322.66	29.35
Texas	335.77	869.19	17.18
Utah	25.13	78.64	20.94
Vermont	24.30	52.33	13.64
Virginia	106.88	300.28	18.79
Washington	138.81	290.57	13.10
West Virginia	26.12	92.92	23.55
Wisconsin	184.28	558.53	20.30
Wyoming	4.04	11.26	18.63
Total U.S.	8,543,000	20,376.34	15.59

SOURCES: See note 2 for the Introduction and Summary in the back of this book.

Note: Both state and federal funds are included. Figures are "provider payments"; administrative expenses would add about 5 percent more. Totals may not add because of rounding. Subsequent tables include territories' spending not shown here.

such welfare-oriented spending have changed since the late 1960s and early 1970s, and spending increases are especially difficult to support (table 2 presents annual rates of increase by year) politically during fiscally troubled times.

Politically, the underlying cost problem seems to be the seemingly unpredictable and nearly uncontrollable nature of Medicaid increases, not merely the absolute level of expenditures in a state. Because Medicaid is a vendor-payment program that buys providers' services, during periods of severe inflation price increases are unavoidable. Because Medicaid is an entitlement program offering free choice of provider (until the 1981 modifications), its rising costs cannot be directly controlled through a fixed budget, rationing, or other managerial means. Thus Medicaid cuts almost always must be achieved by program changes, and these often require legislation and federal approval. Short-term emergency cuts can be much harder to implement than cuts imposed on conventional state operations, for which the main cost is state employees' salaries and wages.

Pressures for Change and State Reactions

The long-run trend of Medicaid spending outpacing revenue growth has often created political support for state restraints on Medicaid—even prior to the Reagan administration and 1981 federal changes. But the states have reacted to the pressures in quite different ways. As Medicaid spending outpaced predictions, many states continued to expand their programs and to pay for continuing price inflation, often through supplemental appropriations partway through a budget period. Other states have taken more or less drastic measures to curb spending. (Chapter 3 details cost-containment strategies used before and after the 1981 changes.) High spending increases by themselves have not necessarily caused problems for the states, however, and low rates have not guaranteed tranquillity. Indeed, Wyoming had an average annual increase of 18.6 percent between 1973 and 1979, yet according to a recent survey that state is unique in expecting no Medicaid deficit and is planning no program changes.[8] The absolute size of Medicaid budgets, the political view taken of Medicaid spending, and the developments on the revenue side of the budget balance are all very important.

Most states seem to have made significant program changes only under severe fiscal pressures. Typically, only some unexpected short-run deficit would shock policymakers into making major cuts. Occasionally, however, policymakers did act to cut spending not because of unpredicted deficits but because political attitudes changed to make predictable long-run increases no longer tolerable. Common precipitating factors for Medicaid crises have been short-term cost overruns or revenue shortfalls during a single budget year (or, in some states, a biennium) which have forced emergency actions to keep budgets in balance.

Overruns can occur for many reasons. Program costs may exceed budgeted amounts because they were underestimated to begin with. Medicaid program officials commonly complain that state legislators intentionally underestimate program spending at budget time, forcing later supplemental appropriations or program changes. (Conversely, legislative sources have argued that these tactics are the only way to pressure Medicaid program managers into holding down spending.) State revenues can also be abruptly curtailed by unexpectedly severe recession, a political "tax revolt" like California's Proposition 13, or other factors. Revenue reductions like these mean that Medicaid growth must be curtailed along with other government programs.

Similarly, budgeted Medicaid savings have often failed to materialize in practice, as when some cost-saving reform falls short of expectations or some unanticipated side effects or reactions to it increase costs elsewhere. Alternatively, Medicaid spending has sometimes simply risen above anyone's expectations, as in Michigan in 1979-1980, when unemployment, particularly in automobile-dependent areas, rose rapidly. Once people had exhausted their private health insurance and other benefits, the welfare rolls grew—Medicaid eligibility along with them. In 1980, California's Medicaid caseload unexpectedly jumped 6.2 percent. The same year an unexpectedly large rise in hospital utilization in Maryland increased costs and necessitated program changes there. Also in 1980, the loss of a reimbursement lawsuit brought by nursing homes in Idaho raised the possibility of a sudden increase in spending there.

The early 1980s may be a watershed period in Medicaid program design. State fiscal problems have been joined by the 1981 act as promoters of longer-term change. As of early calendar 1981, one survey of all the states found that more than half reported "moderate to severe" budgetary difficulties.[9] The most commonly cited reasons were (1) state revenue shortfalls due to (a) economic slowdown, (b) lost federal revenue sharing, and (c) formal limitations on state and local taxes or spending; and (2) Medicaid cost increases due to (a) continuing general and medical cost inflation, (b) rises in welfare caseload because of unemployment, and (c) rises in inpatient hospital utilization. Also important is the increasing mood of governmental austerity throughout much of the country. Many Medicaid programs are thus under considerable pressure to achieve economies, and as of the spring of 1982 almost all programs had been making changes or were seriously considering doing so.

Medicaid crises have occurred periodically in many states, especially during and since the 1974-1975 recession. What is new and striking about the early 1980s is how widespread the problems appear to be. Medicaid difficulties exist in small states and large, in urban and rural areas, in every geographic region; they have hit states with restrictive as well as those with relatively generous programs.

Federal Changes of 1981

On top of these state-level fiscal pressures have come federal cutbacks, begun in earnest during the Reagan administration's budget-cutting effort for FY 1982 and thereafter. The administration charged that the open-ended matching grant feature of the Medicaid program was the source of the program's cost problem because it encouraged excessive generosity and wasteful practices by the states. The administration originally proposed a flat "cap" of 5 percent on the growth of the federal Medicaid share for 1982, plus far greater administrative flexibility for the states to implement cuts and restrictions. A fixed federal contribution would have vastly increased pressures on states to cut their programs. Before, of every extra dollar spent by states 55 cents (on average) came from the federal contribution. With a federal cap, each marginal dollar must come 100 percent from state revenues. This cap would have given great federal "cost control" at the expense of shifting the entire burden of controlling Medicaid spending to the states.

Almost all the states' governors opposed the cap proposal and quite effectively lobbied against it in Congress. The states thought it unfair for them to bear the entire fiscal burden when national economic policy had caused the recession that had virtually eliminated earlier state surpluses by raising expenses and lowering revenues. Moreover, states argued, past and continuing federal policies have contributed to the medical cost inflation that the national government was not taking action to curb, making it impossible for Medicaid programs to curtail their own spending except by dropping people or services from coverage and shifting more burdens to local governments.

Few states believed that increased efficiency under any new flexibility could contribute enough to avoid severe problems. During congressional deliberations on the administration proposals, the Senate favored one alternative, reducing the minimum federal matching percentage from 50 to 40 percent, which would have significantly reduced revenues to twelve states, while the House favored smaller cuts for all states. Both houses of Congress rejected the administration's original proposal.

The Omnibus Budget Reconciliation Act, signed in August 1981, gave the states more money and less administrative flexibility than the president had proposed. Congress nonetheless sent a clear signal to the states that the era of expansion was over. The 1981 act, first applicable to federal FY 1982, beginning in October 1981, calls for future federal Medicaid contributions to be computed as under previous law, but for the dollar contribution in each year to be reduced by a small but increasing percentage; thus the cut will be 3 percent in 1982, 4 percent in 1983, and 4.5 percent in 1984. The federal contribution, however, remains open-ended, and the minimum basic matching percentage is still 50 percent (roughly, 48.5 percent after the 3 percent cut).

The federal reductions can themselves be reduced if states take certain economizing actions. States may offset the reduction dollar-for-dollar for any amount by which they hold FY 1982 spending below a target amount—set at 109 percent of the previously projected FY 1981 level. Future target spending levels will be indexed upward from 109 percent by the medical care component of the consumer price index. Moreover, the 3 percent reduction is itself decreased by one percentage point for states in each of the following circumstances: (a) states which operate approved hospital rate setting-programs, (b) states which have unemployment over 150 percent of the national average, and (c) states which save more than 1 percent of the federal contribution through fraud and abuse recovery programs. The result is a small increase in the already considerable pressure on states to economize. (Another change in FY 1982 federal support occurred automatically, as new federal contribution percentages were computed, based on the most recent income data for states. Some percentages rose and some fell; seldom was the difference as large as the 3 percent cut.)

Congress also directly reduced state and federal Medicaid expenditures by changing certain rules for the treatment of earned income of AFDC recipients; the effect was to reduce eligibility for both AFDC and Medicaid. The eligibility reductions for the AFDC program will be greater than the decline for Medicaid because some of the discontinued AFDC eligibles will continue in Medicaid in states with medically needy programs.

Congress also acted indirectly to promote economizing by giving states somewhat more flexibility to make many kinds of selective efficiencies and targeted cuts in their programs. (Different state cost-containment strategies before and after the 1981 act are considered in more detail in chapter 3.) No cuts were imposed on the program, however, and no mandatory or optional services were dropped from federal assistance. One eligibility category—coverage for those under age twenty-one who do not receive AFDC payments but who would be eligible for AFDC if they attended school—was made optional rather than mandatory. States also are now free to offer different amounts of services to different categories of people in their medically needy programs, although certain restrictions remain (e.g., any plan must cover pregnancy and delivery).

One of the most important 1981 federal changes permits states to pay hospitals differently—not their "reasonable costs" (virtually equivalent to actual spending) but only the amounts needed to finance economical and efficient institutions and to maintain beneficiaries' access to care. This change has the effect of allowing states to reduce their rates for hospital care if they so desire, with considerably less effort than was previously needed to implement a rate-setting program as an "alternative" reimbursement system.

Congress retained the generally "free choice of provider" for the beneficiaries, but allowed states to buy laboratory services and medical devices by competitive bidding and to require physicians and patients to use those low-cost services. Moreover, the Department of Health and Human Services (HHS) received greater authority to grant waivers to states which permit them to restrict the free choice of patients who overuse services; states may pay (only) for cost-effective noninstitutional care, or may exclude from participation in Medicaid providers who overcharge or provide too much care. (Such actions are called a "lock-in" and "lock out," respectively).

This increased flexibility was meant to help states to contain costs just as the reduction in federal matching payments was intended to force states to make difficult spending reductions. Reducing the matching payments increased the cost of each dollar of Medicaid services to each state. However, virtually all states have indicated that the decline in the economy has had greater impact on them than have the federal changes in Medicaid financing procedures.[10] Although the economy's decline is a more significant factor, the reduction in matching payments has had more uniform and consistent influence on state Medicaid policy, since economic conditions among states vary considerably.

CHAPTER 2

DETERMINANTS OF MEDICAID SPENDING

Patterns of Spending Increases

Medicaid spending has from the beginning far outpaced expectations. In 1967 (the program's first full year), total costs were $2.3 billion; by 1975, costs had climbed to $12.3 billion (see table 2). For 1979 (the most recent year for which complete data are available), the total was $20.5 billion, of which the state and local share was $9.9 billion.

While Medicaid spending has risen extremely rapidly ever since its inception, the reasons for the increases have varied. Total spending is always a function of the number of recipients, the volume of services used, and the unit price of services. The relative contributions of these factors to increased spending, however, has varied over time.

In the early years of the program, the number of recipients increased rapidly, as eligibility standards were eased and an increasing proportion of those eligible decided to accept Medicaid support for medical services. (Program statistics report only recipients, not those eligible for but not receiving care.) In this sense, increased spending was intentional (even if its full magnitude had not been anticipated), as the costs of medical services for many poor people were shifted from direct state and local spending to Medicaid reimbursement, and as new services that beneficiaries needed were added. The initial intention was that Medicaid was to be the opening wedge, leading to comprehensive coverage of the poor.

Indeed, coverage grew rapidly. The average compound annual increase in recipients between 1968 and 1973 was 11.7 percent.

TABLE 2

TOTAL FEDERAL AND STATE MEDICAID SPENDING,
FY 1966-1979

Fiscal Year	Payments (In $ millions)	Percentage Increase Over Previous Year
1966	$ 1,592	NA
1967	2,270	42.7
1968	3,451	52.0
1969	4,356	26.1
1970	5,094	17.1
1971	6,345	24.6
1972	7,346	15.8
1973	8,640	15.5
1974	9,983	NA
1975	12,292	23.1
1976	14,135	15.0
1977	16,277	15.2
1978	17,966	10.4
1979	20,474	14.0

SOURCES: See table 1.

Note: Includes Medicaid's predecessor program (Kerr-Mills) between 1966 and 1970.
Figures are "provider payments" which do not include administrative costs
of less than 5 percent. Data reporting changed beginning in 1973.

(Table 7 in chapter 3 supplies the numbers of recipients.) The number of total recipients peaked in 1976; the level in 1979 was actually lower than that in 1974.[1] Unlike the earlier period, then, rapidly higher spending between 1973 and 1979 was *not* due to more lenient eligibility for Medicaid and to growth in the number of people receiving care. To the contrary, most states during the latter part of the 1970s were restricting eligibility standards. Since 1979, the number of recipients has risen and it is projected to peak again in 1982 at about the 1977 level.[2]

Between 1973 and 1979 expenditure increases stemmed mainly from expansions in service coverage and in unit prices. The volume of services used per recipient, or utilization, also seems to have grown somewhat over time for most categories of services. (The *intensity* of services, as well as the absolute *number* provided is important.) Table 3 shows that despite the slight drop in *total* recipients between 1975 and 1979 these increases ranged up to 19 percent (for days in intermediate care facilities—ICFs).

TABLE 3

Utilization of Medicaid Services,
FY 1975 and 1979

	FY 1975	FY 1979	Percentage Change
General hospital inpatient days	34,122,000	35,343,000	+3.6
Intermediate care facility days	157,484,000	187,376,000	+19.0
Skilled nursing days	118,775,000	115,557,000	−2.7
Prescriptions	154,701,000	177,657,000	+14.8

Sources: See table 1.

These increases in utilization probably mainly reflect more intensive use of existing Medicaid services, but they also may reflect a broadening of Medicaid benefits to cover additional services. States have expanded care in intermediate care facilities both to reduce reliance on more expensive skilled nursing facilities (SNFs) and also to bring under Medicaid other facilities that had been providing less skilled nursing and personal care, largely at state expense. This ICF benefit grew rapidly, as table 3 and table 4 both show. In addition, states upgraded "ICF/MRs" (ICFs caring for the mentally retarded) to meet Medicaid certification standards and thereby received federal Medicaid matching funds for Medicaid eligibles. Table 4 demonstrates that these two optional services have been among the fastest-growing items in Medicaid. (The data in tables 3 and 4 cover 1975 and 1979 because utilization data are not uniformly available for previous years.)

The major reason for cost increases, certainly in recent times, is higher prices. Nationwide, increased prices accounted for two-thirds of increased spending on *all* personal health care between 1973 and 1979.[3] Data to calculate a comparable proportion for Medicaid are not available, but price increases are clearly the primary reason for program growth. Unlike expansions in eligibility or service coverage, price increases are *not* politically intended. They are, however, necessary to maintain program coverage of "mainstream" medical care providers in competition with Medicare and private insurers who pay more. Recent cost rises probably are less tolerable politically for this reason than were earlier ones. Nationally, the

TABLE 4

TOTAL MEDICAID PROVIDER PAYMENTS
BY CATEGORY, FY 1975 AND 1979
(In $ millions and percentages)

Category	FY 1975	FY 1979	Average Annual Compound Percentage Increase
Inpatient—general hospital	3,411.4 (27.8)	5,650.7 (27.6)	13.4
Inpatient—mental hospital	399.7 (3.3)	778.0 (3.8)	18.1
Nursing homes			
Skilled nursing facility	2,446.2 (19.9)	3,378.1 (16.5)	8.4
Intermediate care facility/ mentally retarded	348.5 (2.8)	1,515.0 (7.4)	44.4
Intermediate care facility (other)	1,866.7 (15.2)	3,767.0 (18.4)	18.9
Physicians	1,247.7 (10.2)	1,637.9 (8.0)	7.0
Outpatient hospital	377.2 (3.1)	839.4 (4.1)	22.1
Drugs	832.2 (6.8)	1,208.0 (5.9)	9.8
Dental services	349.7 (2.8)	429.9 (2.1)	5.3
Clinics	388.8 (3.2)	266.2 (1.3)	−9.0
All other	624.3 (5.1)	1,003.2 (4.9)	12.6
Total provider payments	$12,292.4 (100.0)	$20,473.5 (100.0)	13.6

SOURCES: See table 1.

interaction of changes in recipients, utilization, and price of services
is illustrated in table 5.

A comparison of the recent period (1973-1979) to the earlier one
(1968-1973) shows the relative importance of the three factors: In
the recent period, growth in total expenditures was 15.6 percent per
year, as the number of recipients increased by 1.2 percent annually,
price increases averaged 9.8 percent, and overall utilization (payment per recipient in constant dollars) rose 4.1 percent. (This com-

TABLE 5

MEDICAID PAYMENTS ADJUSTED FOR CHANGE
IN RECIPIENTS AND PRICES, FY 1968-1979, SELECTED YEARS

Fiscal Year	Total Provider Payments (In $ billions)	Recipients (In millions)	Payments per Recipient (In nominal $)	Medical Care Price Index[a]	Payments per Recipient (In constant $)
1968	3.5	11.5	304	100.0	304
1970	5.1	14.5	351	113.7	309
1973	8.6	20.0	430	129.8	331
1974	10.0	22.0	455	141.9	321
1975	12.3	22.4	549	158.9	346
1976	14.3	24.7	579	174.1	333
1977	16.3	23.8	685	190.8	359
1978	18.0	23.1	779	208.5	374
1979	20.5	21.5	954	226.9	422

Average Annual Compound Rate of Growth (Percent)

1968-1973	+ 19.7	+ 11.7	+ 7.2	+ 5.4	+ 1.7
1973-1979	+ 15.6	+ 1.2	+ 14.2	+ 9.8	+ 4.1

SOURCES: See table 1.

a. Medical care component of the CPI.

putation assumes that price inflation was the same for Medicaid as in other medical services.) Earlier, the 1968-1973 average annual growth rate in spending of 19.7 percent was due more strongly to growth in number of recipients (11.7 percent a year) than to inflation (5.4 percent) or utilization (1.7 percent).

Table 6 gives another view of the importance of recent inflation in health care prices. Since 1973 increases in payments for many services have far outpaced increases in use of services. Of course, patterns vary somewhat by state and by type of provider payments, reflecting differential success in controlling eligibility, use of services, and prices.

Recent Medicaid spending increases have not been constant across different categories of providers, as table 4 showed. Of large expenditure areas, skilled nursing facility care, physician services, drugs, and dental and clinic services have all grown much more slowly than average. The high increases were for care in intermediate care

TABLE 6

GROWTH OF UTILIZATION AND
PAYMENTS FOR SELECTED SERVICES, FY 1973–1979

Service	Average Annual Compound Rate of Growth (Percent)	
	Units of Care	Total Payments
Inpatient hospitals	+2.5	+12.6
Skilled nursing facilities	−1.1	+ 9.0
Intermediate care facilities	+4.3	+17.6
Drugs	+5.6	+11.3

SOURCES: See table 1.

a. ICF data cover 1975 to 1979 only; ICFs were not separately reported in 1973 and 1974.

facilities, including ICF/MRs, mental hospitals, and general hospital outpatient services.

In sum, states have experienced rapid increases in spending, as already noted, averaging 15.6 percent a year between 1973 and 1979, as table 1 showed earlier. The degree to which states have been affected, however, varies with economic factors in the state (e.g., rate of unemployment, population of aged), decisions by the states on the breadth and depth of their Medicaid programs, and the different experiences of the states with cost containment.

This rapid growth needs to be kept in perspective. Despite all the attention paid to spending growth in Medicaid since the mid-1970s, Medicaid's spending rises are not out of line with increases in other health expenditures. Table 5 demonstrated that payments per Medicaid recipient in constant dollars increased only 4.1 percent a year between 1973 and 1979. The increase in medical prices for *all* payers (Medicare, private insurance, and self-payers as well as Medicaid) accounts for most of recent spending rises; much of the rest is due to service shifts, notably to ICFs and ICF/MRs. Another comparison shows that Medicaid spending has risen roughly in step with other spending. Between 1973 and 1979 Medicaid spending rose by 42.3 percent (see table 5), but Medicare spending rose by 62.7 percent, all private health care spending rose 94.8 percent, and the average cost per community hospital inpatient day rose by fully 112.2 percent.[4]

State Choices and Medicaid Spending

The main goal of Medicaid—the reason why states participate and the federal government contributes to their effort—is to buy medical care for lower-income people who meet categorial and medical requirements. Of course, all states are not equally devoted to buying medical care for the poor. How generous to recipients and providers a Medicaid program is designed to be varies with the state's political philosophy and wealth. Some programs are generous in their coverage of potential eligibles and services, yet restrictive in the amounts paid to providers. Others are exactly the reverse. Indeed, there is evidence that most states trade off coverage of people and coverage of benefits.[5]

The first political choice is how much to spend on Medicaid services as opposed to some other public good. The second choice is how to design a structure (within federal requirements) to keep Medicaid entitlements within the desired fiscal bounds. In practice, states must first create a structure, then monitor the results, and finally tinker with the design to make savings. Theoretically, states might control spending through more efficient ways of delivering medical services to the poor, but federal statute has already made the basic choice of the insured, cost-based, fee-for-service system with free choice of provider. Given that (poorly controlled) system, traditionally only very limited room (with federal waivers) has remained for restructuring the delivery system or provider and patient incentives. (The 1981 act has changed these limits somewhat.)

The major determinant of program expense, therefore, is the choice of how generous to be; as was just noted, existing patterns of medical practice and of price inflation then will largely determine actual spending. This choice is very political and state-specific.[6] The Medicaid program in Texas, for example, is stringent on a variety of fronts: By statute, it provides no coverage unless there is federal financial participation, and it covers only a quarter as many people as live below the poverty line (as against 53 percent for the entire nation). Unlike most states, Texas has no medically needy program and covers only thirteen optional services of a possible thirty-two. (Only twelve states cover fewer, while eleven cover twenty-five or more services.) Texas therefore spends a relatively small amount on Medicaid compared with personal income in the state, even though it pays full Medicare rates to hospitals and physicians.

Any high-spending state "could" follow the Texas example and "save" large amounts of Medicaid money.[7] But to the extent that state and local governments end up financing care for uncovered people or services, this may be a false "economy." In any case, most states choose approaches that differ from the approach Texas has taken. What factors then explain the variety of approaches states have chosen and the wide range of generosity shown by their Medicaid programs? The choice of level for initial coverage depends primarily on the state's attitude toward medical care for the poor. Also important is the political climate of welfare, since much Medicaid eligibility is linked to AFDC. Indeed, supporters of broader Medicaid coverage are usually scrupulous in emphasizing the medical nature of Medicaid, while advocates of a narrower program often call it welfare. A state's willingness to support higher Medicaid spending also seems to be associated with high medical costs—and hence the relative need of disadvantaged beneficiaries for assistance. A state's ability to raise revenues is also important: If other factors are equal, states tend to provide relatively higher Medicaid benefits when they have higher levels of personal income and federal support.[8] Particularly in states with a high federal matching percentage, provider interests and state policy may coincide in seeking to maintain a high level of federal contribution to a state's medical economy.

Although political philosophy and available revenues are the chief determinants of how states originally establish and subsequently cut their Medicaid programs, some other factors also play a role. The open-ended nature of the match, whatever the percentage level for a given state, often makes it attractive to substitute Medicaid spending for other state (or local) spending for which the federal match, if any, is less than Medicaid's. This substitution incentive is, of course, strongest in states that have undertaken significant non-Medicaid responsibilities. Perhaps the best example of such substitutions is the optional ICF/MR coverage, of which forty-seven states have taken advantage to help pay for state institutional care for the mentally retarded.[9] Social services (Title XX assistance) and maternal and child health (Title V) are two other areas in which federal dollars are limited, so that marginal spending must be funded entirely with state dollars. It is therefore attractive to switch funding of such services to Medicaid whenever possible as, for example, in the case of transportation for the elderly to get medical care and of prenatal care for welfare mothers.[10]

The same incentive to obtain federal matching dollars also applies to more general care for the poor. States, counties, and cities have always borne a large share of the responsibility for providing care to indigent populations. The need for some level of government to serve as provider or payer of last resort will not disappear if Medicaid eligibility is constrained. A more likely outcome would be a shift in financial responsibility to cities and counties, or perhaps to the state itself, with no accompanying federal matching payments. Broad Medicaid eligibility standards (and higher federal assistance) may thus reduce overall medical spending by states (and its counties and cities) rather than increase it. It is true that a non-Medicaid system for financing or delivering care might be administered so as to cost less than combined state-federal Medicaid—if beneficiaries were prevented from receiving as much care, if providers were paid less per unit (and hence would deliver a different quality of care or mix of services), or if the same care could be provided more efficiently. In the extreme case, a non-Medicaid regime might prefer to deter some people from seeking public assistance at all. (This is really a judgment that some Medicaid services are not worth their cost.) Such "efficiencies," if such they are, would have to be truly enormous to compensate for the loss of 55 percent federal matching (on average). Although states want to achieve some such "efficiencies," totally abandoning federal aid to do so is very unattractive.

The importance of federal requirements in shaping state Medicaid programs (and any cuts made in them) can hardly be overstated. Traditionally, federal law has established the basic design of Medicaid as an entitlement program, with mandatory benefits, offering full access to care with free choice of provider and generally cost-based provider reimbursement. A host of lesser requirements has further reduced the states' own freedom of choice under Medicaid, although the 1981 act has considerably increased state flexibility. All these factors make Medicaid costs extremely hard to predict or control and probably increase the amount that states spend over what they might choose to spend without restrictions.

The existence of federal requirements also provides additional, nonstate forums for interests affected by Medicaid policy, one of which is Congress. For example, nursing home payment policy before the mid-1970s was left almost entirely to the states, which were often very restrictive. The situation was then radically altered by a new federal mandate for "reasonably cost-related" reimbursement, which was itself modified in 1980 to permit greater state discretion. Another forum is the federal courts, which must often interpret rather vague federal provisions. These interpretations affect states' abilities to set eligibility standards, benefit coverage, payment methods, and regulatory policy.

The relative political influence of provider and beneficiary interests is also important. Sometimes provider and recipient interests are allied, other times they are not. In "normal" times of traditional program expansion, beneficiary and provider constituencies pulled in the same direction—toward good coverage and full payment—but budgetary pressures can force states to choose between the two. States vary considerably in the extent to which they will squeeze providers to avoid cutting beneficiaries' eligibility or services, or vice versa. Different provider groups also fare quite differently. Once again, this phenomenon underlines the political nature of such choices.

All these factors have helped to shape state Medicaid choices, both the initial scope of program chosen and the multitudinous shifts undertaken since, both to expand and contract spending. Ultimately, achieving cost savings becomes the inverse of the original construction of a Medicaid program; it is principally a matter of political choice of how much to provide and what a state can afford.

State Medicaid programs have usually been unwilling to watch their expenditures grow without limit. Since the mid-1970s they have identified and enforced literally hundreds of economies, small and large. The first major wave of Medicaid program cutbacks came in the mid-1970s in reaction to the economic recession of 1974–1975. The late 1970s, in contrast, were a time of modest program growth in almost all states. Earlier cuts were often restored, new services were added, and other liberalizations adopted, although many times against a backdrop of improved administration and tightened enforcement of existing rules.

Amidst the welter of Medicaid program detail, one simple conclusion about past state behavior is probably most striking: despite strong and growing budgetary pressure, by dint of very inventive program shifts and juggling, almost no state has significantly retreated from the scope of its original Medicaid program. Although Medicaid is totally voluntary, all states have elected to participate (Arizona only recently, on a limited, demonstration basis), and no state has dropped out. Moreover, states' devotion to whatever level of beneficiary and service coverage they have chosen is marked. As the next chapter will describe, large cuts in eligibility or services covered are the last ways used to save program dollars. States typically turn first to supplemental appropriations and fiscal juggling, such as postponing expenditures. Historically, Medicaid programs have preferred administrative streamlining, crackdowns on errors and abuses, expanded collections from third parties, relatively small economies, and "Band Aid" measures to scaling back their total effort under Medicaid (and thus also their federal match). Some states have tried hard to reduce provider fees and payments, but few have drastically cut eligibility and services as a result of fiscal pressures. One explanation is that states had good reasons for establishing the types of Medicaid coverage that they did, so the states tend to change only that coverage incrementally, if such a course is at all possible. Another explanation is that very few states (until very recently) have faced enough sustained fiscal pressure to force major changes.

Many program cuts between the mid-1970s and the early 1980s were made hastily, under great political pressure to save money (or at least state Medicaid program dollars) in the same or next budgetary period. Such pressure put a premium on "quick fixes" rather than major structural change for a long-term solution. Medicaid decision makers may thus have acted hastily without being able to consider the likely side effects of particular Medicaid cuts on other state spending—whether under Medicaid itself or in other parts of a state's budget. In the past the cuts may have been made in ignorance of their effects or with the expectation that the cuts would soon be rescinded as unemployment eased or state revenues increased.

Greater experience with the effects of cuts and more sophisticated Medicaid management have improved understanding of the dynamics of program redesign for cost containment, and long-term fiscal stringency has increased in many states and at the federal level. Future cuts are more apt to be carefully considered for their long-term effects.

CHAPTER 3

STATE COST-CONTAINMENT STRATEGIES, BEFORE AND AFTER 1981 CHANGES

Despite federal requirements, states have always had considerable discretion in establishing the general structure of their programs as well as in making specific adjustments to contain state spending.[1] The changes in federal requirements made by the 1981 Omnibus Budget Reconciliation Act increased the states' discretion. This chapter discusses how states have traditionally acted to constrain spending and how the 1981 act's changes have been implemented.

The number of policy choices affecting spending in a given Medicaid program—regardless of whether they have ever been ever explicitly decided upon—is enormous. Policymakers seeking to trim (or expand) programs confront a truly staggering array of options, ranging from changing an administrative interpretation of a single eligibility rule to dropping out of the program altogether.

There are four main categories of change to consider. The first three are the components of the spending equation—spending equals recipients times utilization times price:

1. *Eligibility* is what the state can more or less directly control in attempting to curtail the number of people receiving Medicaid services. A state cannot limit the absolute number of eligibles according to its fiscal situation, but it can set Medicaid and welfare eligibility standards expected to achieve a certain result. Because Medicaid eligibility entitles each beneficiary to determine whether to seek medical attention, determining actual recipients is beyond direct state control.

2. *Service coverage and utilization* consist of the scope and duration of benefits covered under Medicaid, plus the use that beneficiaries make of them. Although many services must be covered,

23

many are optional, and a significant part of a program's scope is within the state's discretion. Again, because Medicaid is an entitlement program, the actual use the beneficiaries make of covered services can be affected only indirectly, through various authorization, review, and control procedures.

3. *Provider payment* discretion is rather extensive, although the states' ability to set payment rules varies for different types of providers.

4. *Other measures* include all the administrative steps that states may also take to save money, as well as major innovations in program approach such as prepayment for care and provision of alternatives to institutional long-term care. Within each category, we first discuss the states' traditional options, and then the changes introduced in 1981 (and first applicable to FY 1982). Our purposes are to explain the difficulty of making significant reductions in the program, to explore the possible side effects of contractions in some detail, and to analyze the likely effects of the new "flexibility" in the Medicaid statute.

To gain some understanding of the implementation and effects of the 1981 Medicaid policy changes made by Congress and the Reagan administration, we contacted Medicaid and budget officials in ten important states during March and April 1982. In five states, Connecticut, Florida, Maryland, New York, and Pennsylvania, officials envisaged few significant changes in Medicaid for FY 1982, and only Maryland officials expected to stay within the 109 percent target. One possible reason is that tight controls, particularly on hospital payment, had been in place for several years in each state except Pennsylvania. Another is that two of the states had experienced increases in their matching rates in FY 1982 because their average per capita income relative to the national average had declined. In New York, the federal matching rate increased from 50.0 to 50.9 percent and in Pennsylvania from 55.1 to 56.8 percent. For these two states, these increases substantially offset the effect of the 1981 act's reduced federal assistance. Probably more important, however, the decline in economic activity was less severe in these states than in many other parts of the country.

The other five states in which we contacted Medicaid and budget officials—California, Illinois, Kentucky, Michigan, and Oregon— were substantially reducing their programs. In three of these states, (California, Michigan, and Oregon), legislation to limit taxes or expenditures had recently been enacted, while in the other two, (Kentucky and Oregon), Medicaid had recently grown rapidly. Moreover, each of these states had been severely affected by the recession. According to a recent survey of the National Governors Association, several other states that have been hard hit by the recession also are making extensive program changes. These include Wisconsin, Iowa, Missouri, Georgia, and Washington.

Eligibility

Because the amount a Medicaid program spends is most influenced by the number and types of people it covers, cutting eligibility is probably the most powerful way to reduce spending (and, of course, federal contributions to care for those people). Medicaid eligibility rules, which are extremely complex, are only summarized here.[2] If states are to receive any federal payments, they must cover some eligibles, called "categorically eligible" people—those who receive welfare cash assistance, that is, Aid to Families with Dependent Children or Supplemental Security Income. In addition, states may choose to cover other people for whom they also receive federal matching payments. The "optionally categorically eligibles" include people eligible for but not receiving cash welfare assistance. A more important optional group is the "medically needy," persons whose incomes or assets are too high to allow them to receive welfare payments but who still are deemed unable to afford their medical bills. (Medically needy coverage allows people to "spend down" their incomes by incurring medical bills sufficient to reduce their income to welfare levels or a specified percentage above those levels.) As of December 1980, thirty-four states covered the medically needy. Finally, states may include any group they wish entirely at state expense. Many states include persons receiving cash payments under a totally *state* welfare program like General Assistance or Home Relief. Typical "state only" eligibles are able-bodied people between the ages of twenty-one and sixty-five who earn or own enough to handle their basic needs but not enough to meet medical expenses.

There are two main ways to affect Medicaid eligibility, either (1) to control eligibility in the underlying welfare categories or (2) to restrict groups covered specifically and optionally under Medicaid itself. The principal way that states have restricted the number of welfare recipients is through their control over the amount of income and assets people may have and still receive AFDC. States varied widely in their initial generosity, and changes have occurred over time. Most states have failed to raise welfare standards to keep pace with general inflation. As poor people's incomes and assets have risen, more and more have surpassed the eligibility ceilings, dropped off the welfare rolls, and hence lost their Medicaid eligibility. Comparatively few states have even purported to "index" welfare levels to keep up with inflation; states experiencing budgetary crisis are especially likely to hold down increases in welfare ceilings, at least temporarily. In extreme cases, some states, including New Jersey and New York, went for many years with no changes whatsoever in welfare standards. More subtly, changes can be made in the amounts of "income disregards" (items such as work-related expenses that are not counted as income) or of protected assets (those that welfare recipients may retain without affecting eligibility). With respect to aged, blind, or disabled people, states have had less discretion to hold down payment levels arbitrarily since the 1972 federal Social Security Act Amendments and the shift to a more federalized SSI system.

In addition, certain optional welfare groups—such as pregnant women whose children when born will make them eligible for AFDC, and families with unemployed fathers—may simply be dropped from welfare and Medicaid coverage. (These groups may also be covered only for Medicaid and not for AFDC as well. In that case, they may simply be dropped from Medicaid coverage.)

States may directly cut optional Medicaid eligibles, including people who are eligible for welfare but do not receive it, people who would be eligible for welfare if they were not institutionalized in a hospital or nursing home, and all children under age twenty-one who are financially eligible (who thus need not be categorically eligible). In addition, a state may change medically needy eligibility standards (e.g., by reducing from 33 percent to 10 percent the amount by which the income of Medicaid beneficiaries may surpass welfare cash-assistance limits), or it may drop medically needy coverage altogether.

During and since the recessionary "crunch" of the mid-1970s, many states have cut eligibility in one or more of these ways. Some optional eligibility groups, like unemployed parents, are frequently cut. State-only eligibles (who receive no federal funding) are especially likely to be targeted for cuts. States generally have not cut optional groups such as people who would be eligible for welfare if they applied (because to do so would simply force them to apply) or people in institutions who would become eligible outside (since it is politically distasteful and legally difficult to attempt to evict from a nursing home a dependent person who would then become a welfare burden in any case).

Low welfare levels create low medically needy standards as well because the latter may not exceed 133.33 percent of the former. Moreover, outright reductions in medically needy standards are not unheard of; in Michigan, for example, the legislature rolled back the percentage from 120 to 110 in 1975. Several states are now considering stronger measures to curb the medically needy population, up to and including abolition of coverage (and the 1981 act increased state discretion here, as will be seen). Despite the relatively high cost of serving the medically needy, no state that has once established medically needy coverage has subsequently abolished it.

In general, taking direct action that affects existing beneficiaries is much less popular than is relying on inflation to make cuts. Not only are direct cuts more visible, but they also require formal advance notice to the group being cut. Moreover, poverty lawyers have been reasonably successful in blocking or delaying group cuts for failure to comply with federal regulations. Probably the most important constraint on eligibility reductions is the fact that many of the medically needy are elderly and institutionalized. As a result, elimination of eligibility would be extremely unpopular politically. In addition, eligibility cutbacks affecting people who are not institutionalized will often result in a shift of financial burden to county-run hospitals and clinics and ultimately to local taxpayers. Inherent in any such shift is the loss of federal matching payments.

Since the mid-1970s the number of Medicaid recipients has actually declined, as table 5 showed. Restrictive state policies have doubtless played a role. It appears that, relative to the number of poor people, Medicaid protection declined during the 1970s. The ratio of Medicaid recipients to the below-poverty-line population dropped from 0.59 in 1970 to 0.53 in 1979. Table 7 gives state-by-state comparisons. (Note: Existing statistics do not show what *percentage* of poor people receive Medicaid. Some Medicaid recipients are not below the poverty line, for example, the medically needy for whom high medical bills reduce their incomes to Medicaid levels. But the *ratio* of recipients to the poverty population is still a good measure of medical coverage relative to the needy population.)

TABLE 7

RATIO OF MEDICAID RECIPIENTS TO PERSONS
LIVING BELOW THE POVERTY LEVEL, BY STATE, FY 1970 AND 1979

State	FY 1970	FY 1979
Massachusetts	—[a]	1.15
Hawaii	0.95	0.94
California	1.74	0.93
Rhode Island	0.96	0.92
New York	1.56	0.79
District of Columbia	0.91	0.72
Maine	0.44	0.71
Pennsylvania	0.93	0.69
Puerto Rico	—[a]	0.68
Oregon	0.38	0.67
Maryland	0.76	0.66
New Jersey	0.55	0.64
Michigan	0.54	0.58
Wisconsin	0.59	0.58
Alaska	—[b]	0.57
Illinois	0.55	0.55
U.S. TOTAL—AVERAGE	0.59	0.53
Connecticut	0.75	0.53
Delaware	0.61	0.52
Washington	0.84	0.51
Minnesota	0.57	0.47
Kentucky	0.43	0.46
Vermont	0.71	0.44
Kansas	0.45	0.43
Louisiana	0.23	0.42
Oklahoma	0.46	0.42
Colorado	0.61	0.40
Ohio	0.36	0.40
Alabama	0.17	0.39
New Hampshire	0.45	0.39
Iowa	0.36	0.37
South Carolina	0.16	0.37
Utah	0.46	0.37
Virginia	0.21	0.35
Arkansas	0.10	0.34
Missouri	0.38	0.34
Tennessee	0.19	0.33
Montana	0.28	0.32
Wyoming	0.19	0.32
Georgia	0.35	0.31
Idaho	0.27	0.30
New Mexico	0.28	0.30
North Carolina	—[a]	0.30

TABLE 7 (continued)

State	FY 1970	FY 1979
Indiana	0.24	0.29
Mississippi	0.16	0.26
Nevada	0.44	0.26
West Virginia	0.35	0.26
Florida	0.27	0.24
Nebraska	0.33	0.24
North Dakota	0.24	0.24
South Dakota	0.17	0.24
Texas	0.18	0.24

SOURCES: See table 1.

    a. Information unavailable for at least one of the factors—population, low-income population, or Medicaid recipients.

    b. No Medicaid recipients in 1970.

The disparity among the states has lessened in this time; the spread in 1970 was from 0.10 to 1.74, whereas in 1979 the range was 0.24 to 1.15. Moreover, all thirteen states at or above the 1970 average of 0.59 percent reduced their ratio by 1979. Of those below average in 1970, twenty-one increased, eleven decreased, and two were unchanged. This pattern seems to indicate greater tightening of eligibility in states that had initially been generous.

The 1981 act made a number of changes in eligibility. The most important were these:

1. States were required to limit expenses counted against income in determining eligibility for AFDC grants; this policy reduces the numbers of AFDC, and thus Medicaid, eligibles.

2. Coverage of persons under age twenty-one who do not receive AFDC payments, but who would be eligible for AFDC if they were in school, became optional rather than mandatory.

3. States were prohibited from making cash-assistance payments to first-time pregnant women until the sixth month of pregnancy; states were given the option of providing AFDC benefits thereafter. (They also retained the option of providing Medicaid benefits from the time pregnancy was medically verified.)

4. Medically needy income and asset levels were permitted to vary between groups (e.g., aged vs. disabled). This change allows states to target additional optional coverage more selectively.

In addition, through a provision in the 1980 Omnibus Budget Reconciliation Act that was not implemented until late in FY 1981, states were permitted to exclude from eligibility people who "impoverished" themselves by giving away assets to qualify for medical assistance (for example, giving a home to children before entering a nursing home). Technically, the new rule allows a presumption that, if during the two years prior to applying for Medicaid coverage, an applicant has transferred assets to someone else and received less than fair market value in exchange, that person may be presumed to have done so to establish Medicaid eligibility. If the applicant cannot rebut this presumption, she or he may be denied Medicaid coverage.

All states are required to implement the AFDC cutbacks mandated by the 1981 act. Officials in states with medically needy programs generally did not expect these cuts to have a significant impact because the same persons who were cut from AFDC could become eligible for Medicaid as medically needy (or, rarely, under state-only assistance). Yet to qualify as medically needy, people will have to "spend down" some of their own income before their Medicaid coverage begins. Some savings will therefore result, but the amount is uncertain. For example, Michigan reported that AFDC eligibility fell between January 1981 and January 1982 by some 35,000 persons, while medically needy rolls increased by only about 7,000. To the contrary, between the first quarter of 1981 and the first quarter of 1982 Pennsylvania reported a drop of 9,078 AFDC recipients, but an increase of 10,834 in medically needy recipients. Other factors are surely at work as well.

Most of the states we contacted in 1982 (including California, Illinois, Michigan, New York, and Pennsylvania) had made only small increases in AFDC benefit levels or none at all, thus allowing inflation to raise earnings of employed welfare recipients above the eligibility ceilings. Several states, including Alabama, Connecticut, Illinois, Florida, Georgia, North Carolina, and South Carolina, specifically eliminated people between the ages of eighteen and twenty-one. Many other states, including Maryland and Michigan, did not. Eliminating this age group is a minor shift, since the number of people in it is relatively small and their use of medical care relatively light.

Some states, such as California and Washington, reduced their medically needy coverages by increasing the amount that recipients must "spend down" before Medicaid eligibility begins. Since medically needy eligibility levels in most states are tied to AFDC payment standards, the Medicaid levels will also be affected by any limits on the welfare payments. Thus, several states have slowed growth in their medically needy programs by freezing AFDC payments. At the same time, New Jersey and Florida are reported to be considering adding medically needy programs; the 1981 act permits more limited medically needy programs than were previously allowed.

According to surveys by the National Governors Association, several states—including Alabama, Kentucky, Minnesota, Mississippi, Nevada, New Jersey and Washington—have added coverage of pregnant women. One intent of the 1981 legislation was to permit states to provide Medicaid benefits to pregnant women who were no longer receiving cash assistance. Several states reported that they added the benefit because of concern over the future financial consequences of failure to cover high-risk pregnancies.

The transfer-of-assets provision may prove quite important. In the past, people likely to enter nursing homes have sometimes given their assets to their relatives in order to become poor enough to meet Medicaid eligibility requirements. Prior to enactment of the new law, federal courts had effectively prevented states from excluding persons who so transferred their assets from coverage, although a number of states tried to exclude them. The results of tighter standards will be fewer admissions to nursing homes, greater use of these assets to pay for care, or both. A large number of states reported tightening their transfer-of-assets provisions.

In sum, most states have reduced eligibility in FY 1982 , but typically the cuts have not been drastic, and there have been some eligibility increases. Two important exceptions to past practices can be attributed to the 1980 and 1981 Reconciliation Acts: First, the mandated AFDC reductions eliminated some working persons from welfare eligibility and thereby from Medicaid; as noted, many of these people (especially those with significant health problems) are expected to become eligible through medically needy programs. The extent of savings thus achieved is unclear. Second, the tightening of transfer-of-asset requirements will reduce nursing home expenditures; the amount of the savings is again uncertain.

The major constraints on state eligibility reductions continue to apply. States fear the political consequences of reductions in coverage of the institutionalized medically needy, many of whom are elderly and all of whom are quite vulnerable. For many, there is no decent and humane alternative to Medicaid support in a nursing home. With respect to acute services for Medicaid recipients not in long-term institutions, cuts in eligibility may simply shift costs of care because such people do have alternatives: They may be treated in private hospitals which shift costs to private insurers and other payers or (more likely) in public hospitals and clinics, whose deficits are borne by local taxpayers, sometimes with state aid. In either case, federal matching funds are lost to the state economy. Thus, from the state's perspective, eligibility reductions may not be cost-effective, even though they conserve Medicaid dollars.

Services Covered and Utilization Controls

Medicaid benefits (the services covered) are often altered in the interest of economizing. Like Medicaid eligibles, services come in two main categories—mandatory and optional. The mandatory category includes inpatient and outpatient hospital, skilled nursing facility (SNF), and physician services. In addition, states may choose to cover other services. Optional services include intermediate care facilities for both the mentally retarded (ICF/MRs) and all others (ICFs), drugs, and dental care. The federal government shares the cost for all these services. States may cover still more services if they want, but without federal assistance. A state may limit the scope or duration of any service so long as reasonable access to care is preserved, and states need not provide the same coverage for the medically needy as for the categorically eligible.

The services that states cover under Medicaid vary less than do the states' eligibility standards. Covered optional services vary by state.[3] Almost all states covered both types of ICFs and drugs; indeed, these were major expenditures for their Medicaid programs (about one-third of spending, nationwide). At least half the states covered most other optional services. Limitations on service coverage are probably the most common short-range cost-control devices adopted by states seeking to balance their Medicaid budgets. In a crunch, states usually drop coverage of minor optional services altogether—such as chiropractic, podiatric, nonemergency dental, and optical services. (Of course, many jurisdictions never covered these services in the first place.) Major optional categories, however, are seldom affected. In particular, no state has yet dropped ICF or ICF/MR coverage, although they are optional and account for over a quarter of all Medicaid spending. (Texas, however, has recently realigned its ICF/MR definitions to exclude some facilities that had formerly been included.)

Restrictions and limitations on services are allowed for both mandatory and optional services. (For optional services only, recipients may also be required to make nominal copayments.)

The most significant limitation imposed is upon length of stay in a general hospital. Roughly half the states now have such limits, either per admission or per year. Several states apply more specialized limits, such as bans on nonemergency weekend hospital admissions, limitations of pre-operative hospital stays to one day, and exclusion of inpatient surgical procedures that can be performed on an outpatient basis. Physician and other services may also be limited by number of visits per time period or by type. Other common limitations include three outpatient drug prescriptions per month, small copayments for nonemergency ambulance services, a limitation of eyeglasses to one pair per year, and the like. Whether a given limit overly restricts access often has to be tested in court, since the federal law and regulations are not precise on this point.

In contrast to fixed limits, discretionary review to limit coverage to "needed" services is very appealing: Prior authorization, that is, advance approval from a Medicaid reviewer, is commonly required for admission to nursing homes, nonemergency hospital stays, use of out-of-state hospitals, and cosmetic surgery. Sometimes reauthorization is required after a given period. After-the-fact "utilization review" of the necessity for institutional services and the level of care that is provided is also a very attractive cost-control strategy, since it seems to offer savings at no cost in reduced benefits. Administratively, of course, defining, finding, and eliminating inappropriate care can be very difficult and expensive indeed.[4]

Another utilization limitation that is appearing with increasing frequency is the restriction of certain Medicaid recipients found to be high users of service to a single provider or a small number of service providers, such as physicians or pharmacists. This "lock-in" strategy may be coupled with efforts to educate the beneficiaries to use services more appropriately. (The 1981 act approved further expansions in the use of this strategy, as noted later.)

The ebb and flow of Medicaid service limitations since 1975 defy easy categorization and empirical analysis. In general, review requirements are preferred to inflexible limits, restrictions on optional services (and those to the medically needy) are preferred to mandatory services limits, and limitations on individual providers are preferred to limitations on hospitals. Individual providers other than physicians often are even dropped entirely from coverage. Overall, states more often impose limits on services than limits on groups of eligibles.

Over time, the institution of such limits and cuts has varied. Many curbs were imposed during and in the aftermath of the mid-1970s recession. Often, but not always, these were only temporary, being rescinded within a few months or a year. In the later half of the 1970s, most states actually added slightly to benefit coverage, even beyond restoration of previous cuts. A major addition is ICF/MR coverage, which a number of states have added since 1975; by 1980 forty-seven jurisdictions covered ICF/MRs. Because ICF/MRs are usually state institutions,[5] shifting them to Medicaid increases the federal match available to fund them. Smaller benefit increases, such as psychiatric hospital coverage for persons under age twenty-one and ambulatory surgical centers, were not uncommon. An unpublished Health Care Financing Administration (HCFA) analysis of Medicaid state plan amendments between July 1978 and June 1980 revealed that there were more than twice as many increases in services offered (eighty-nine) as decreases (forty). Moreover, the survey found that state plan increases tended to be in major optional service categories such as ICF/MRs, while decreases were in relatively minor categories such as podiatric and chiropractic services.[6]

It should be noted that most of the benefit expansions in recent years were intended to save state money. The psychiatric hospital benefit, like the one for ICF/MR, makes federal matching funds available to help pay for care previously financed almost wholly by the state. Coverage of ambulatory surgery centers is intended to reduce state outlays for hospital inpatient care. The corollary is that benefit cutbacks in these areas would probably increase costs for states.

The 1981 act made these three notable changes in service coverage and utilization:

1. States were permitted to limit services for some but not for all medically needy persons (e.g., to cover dental services for medically needy children, but not for adults).

2. States were permitted to limit freedom of choice (as previously understood) (a) to enter into competitive-bidding arrangements for buying laboratory services or medical supplies and (b) to "lock in" overutilizing recipients or to "lock out" providers who have been found to give too many services or poor quality care—provided reasonable access to care for beneficiaries is maintained. (Other

freedom of choice restrictions on available providers or services are possible by waiver.)

3. Review of Medicaid services by Professional Standards Review Organizations (PSROs) is no longer required; states can contract with PSROs or perform their own review of hospital or long-term-care stays.

States were *not* given any additional freedom to apply copayments on mandatory services for the categorically needy, except through limited waiver authority.

Despite the lack of major changes in their authority, states since enactment of the 1981 legislation have been fairly active in reducing service coverage, presumably because fiscal pressures and the political atmosphere demanded it. Several states began applying limits (or increasing existing limits) on hospital days. Georgia, for example, limited hospital coverage to twenty inpatient days per recipient per year, limited the number of preoperative days prior to elective surgery to one, and ceased coverage of nonemergency weekend admissions. Iowa stopped payment for inpatient care for surgical procedures that could be performed on an outpatient basis; the state also limited reimbursements for inpatient hospital care to the fiftieth percentile for the recipient's diagnosis. Other states (Illinois, Massachusetts, Michigan, Missouri, Rhode Island, South Carolina, and Virginia) applied or are moving to begin applying similar limits—reducing the number of covered days, eliminating weekend admissions, reducing the coverage of preoperative days, and ending payment for inpatient surgery when the service could be provided on an outpatient basis.

Few states are directly limiting physician visits. Several—including California, Connecticut, Illinois, New Jersey, North Carolina, and Pennsylvania—are starting or expanding programs for "locking in" patients who are regarded as "overutilizers." Other states, including Connecticut, Michigan, and Washington, have introduced "second opinion" programs for surgery.

In response to the 1981 act, a number of states are considering bulk purchase arrangements for various goods (e.g., eyeglasses) and some services (e.g., laboratory services). The objective is to buy from the lowest bidder (or at the lowest-bid price) rather than to reimburse every retail seller at its own price. Before 1981, a few states had such arrangements for eyeglasses, hearing aids, and certain durable medical equipment. By federal administrative interpretation, such restrictions were held not to deny freedom of choice. Professional services were more problematic. New York lost a landmark court case, which ruled that its plan for volume purchase of lab tests did indeed limit freedom of choice and was therefore only permissible under a limited demonstration-project waiver. The 1981 act greatly expanded state authority by explicitly providing that bulk purchase of durable medical equipment, lab tests, and X-ray services is indeed consistent with beneficiaries' free choice of provider and therefore needs no waiver. As of spring 1982, many states were planning to add such arrangements, including Alabama, Connecticut, Iowa, Kansas, Michigan, New Jersey, North Dakota, and Washington. As noted, some such arrangements, particularly for supplies, were already in place. For example, Minnesota had already begun developing bulk purchasing of eyeglasses, hearing aids, and durable medical equipment. Michigan and Washington had begun the bulk purchasing of eyeglasses.

Several states are adding controls on the number of nursing home days they will pay for (in either skilled nursing or intermediate care facilities). California, South Dakota, and West Virginia have limited the number of reserved bed days in nursing homes (days in which the patient is at home or otherwise out of the nursing home) they will pay for. Colorado, Connecticut, Kansas, Minnesota, and Utah began statewide screening of patients before admission. Mississippi limited the number of beds for which its program would pay. Wisconsin has requested a waiver to cease paying for the two lowest levels of intermediate care facilities.

Approximately twenty states (including Florida, Georgia, Illinois, Massachusetts, Michigan, Missouri, and Wisconsin) applied or extended limits on drug coverage. These limits involved tightening the drug formulary to restrict the number and kinds of drugs covered, adopting lock-in arrangements for overusers, eliminating over-the-counter drugs, requiring use of generic drugs, limiting the number of drugs per month, and imposing copayments on prescriptions.

Several limits were placed on smaller optional services—services by dentists, chiropractors, podiatrists, optometrists, and the like. Some services were eliminated altogether, while others were limited to certain beneficiaries or made subject to copayments. Copayments have become increasingly important; California, Illinois, Iowa, and Michigan, in particular, have introduced copayments for large numbers of services. Many other states have expressed interest in copayments as a mechanism for controlling costs, particularly if the federal statute were changed to allow copayments on mandatory services (now possible only by waiver). Governors have often complained that they cannot use copayments as much as they would like, and the Reagan administration agrees. Congress has not yet enacted such authority, but it is seriously being considered for FY 1983.

Several states—including California, Georgia, Maryland, Michigan, and Pennsylvania—have moved toward their own review of hospital claims to replace that done by PSROs.

Of all the changes that have been described, the limits on hospital stays are probably the most important. Hospital days are expensive, and it is easier to impose limits on them than to design a new payment system. Alternatively, limits or the threat of limits can be used, as they have been in Illinois, to make hospitals amenable to lower payment rates. Limits are, however, arbitrary and unrelated to needed lengths of care. Thus in many cases, such limits simply transfer costs elsewhere for days that must be given to patients. If Medicaid simply stops paying after fourteen hospital days, for instance, the hospital itself must meet the cost of any further needed care. A private hospital giving such charity care must raise other rates; more likely, public hospitals will have to provide charity when private ones find ways to avoid taking patients who are likely to have long stays. To the extent that limits on hospital days increase public hospital deficits, local taxpayers must ultimately pay, with no federal share. Moreover, the effect of the limit on hospital days varies with the amount of specialty (longer-term) care a hospital gives. Maryland, for example, has found it necessary to provide relief to certain hospitals that provide specialized services.

Provider Payment Policies

By federal law, state Medicaid payment rates must be high enough to attract sufficient providers to make services available to the Medicaid population to the same extent as they are available to the population at large. In addition, providers must accept Medicaid payments as payments in full. Finally, Medicaid payments may not exceed what Medicare and private payers pay for the same service. (In fact, because of economies that states have made, Medicaid payments are almost always lower—with the predictable result of reduced access to mainstream care.)

Within these very general requirements, states have always had some discretion in setting payment levels. States have had the least discretion for inpatient hospital and nursing home care and the most for individual providers (e.g., physicians, druggists, opticians) and hospital outpatient services. States' control over hospital rates was greatly increased by the 1981 act. The most important developments concern hospitals, nursing homes, and physicians.

Inpatient Hospital Care

Traditionally, payments for inpatient hospital service have not been an important target for Medicaid cost containment despite the fact that they have accounted for almost a third of provider payments, as table 4 showed. Under federal law before 1981, states were permitted only two basic methods to pay hospitals: The more commonly used method was Medicare-style "reasonable cost" reimbursement, which offers little control over hospital spending because (with minor exceptions) it means paying the full costs at which each hospital delivers services to Medicaid recipients. Full costs are retroactively determined under various accounting and other rules of allocation. In practice, almost all costs actually incurred by hospitals have been reimbursed, and cost increases have been very hard to control.

In the past, major efforts to control hospital spending were possible only under the second form of Medicaid payment—called the "alternative method" (to Medicare) or state "rate setting"[7] (sometimes also undertaken experimentally under different federal authority). Such programs have varied enormously in complexity and in focus, but all of them attempt to make institutions accept a state's budget rather than the other way around.[8]

Since the early 1970s, alternative methods of payment have been permissible with special HHS approval from the Department of Health and Human Services, first under regulatory interpretation of federal statute, then by statutory amendment. A consensus is developing that rate setting is effective in lowering the rate of increase in hospital spending by several percentage points a year— at least in mature rate-setting programs, after an initial start-up period.[9] But states have been slow to adopt rate setting. Before the 1981 act, only thirteen Medicaid programs had approved alternative systems, two of them only approved in July 1981. (These states did, however, account for a high proportion of total Medicaid spending.) Table 8 shows these states.

There are good reasons for the slow spread of rate setting. Perhaps the most obvious is that rate setting offers no quick or easy solution to rising hospital spending. Many doubted that rate setting could work, at least in their states. Moreover, developing an alternative system that met pre-1981 federal requirements (essentially, one that squeezed hospital revenues but not so much that payment was no longer reasonable) was a lengthy and arduous process in itself, as was winning federal approval and implementing the new system once approved. Quicker, simple limits on percentage increases in per diem hospital payments were tried and abandoned in the mid-1970s after California and Massachusetts lost lawsuits in lower courts on the ground that such arbitrary limits were contrary to federal statute.[10] Such litigation points up another disincentive—frequent rate-setting lawsuits, which not only increase a program's cost but also can significantly delay its effects.[11]

Moreover, rate setting for Medicaid along may not be sufficient to contain spending while maintaining access. Since Medicaid provides only about one-tenth of total hospital revenues, changing its payment method does not materially affect the incentives of most hospitals to increase costs. Reducing only Medicaid rates may simply cause costs to be shifted to other payers or service to Medicaid beneficiaries to be cut. But a broader rate-setting program increases political resistance and may be feared ultimately to reduce medical standards of care.

Stringent rate setting also, by design, hurts hospitals. Their revenue growth and ability to raise capital funds may be considerably curtailed. A number of hospitals in New York have closed their doors under state pressure, and others have, with some success, pressed for various government "bail-outs" to keep operating. Public hospitals may be especially hard hit for two reasons: They serve a disproportionate number of Medicaid patients to begin with, and they are apt to get even more poor patients under stringent Medicaid-only rate setting, since other hospitals may find ways to reduce their Medicaid census. Since local taxpayers finance deficits of public hospitals, one result of this rate setting can be a shift of costs to lower levels of government, with an accompanying loss of federal matching payments. Finally, hospitals are typically far more powerful politically than welfare and Medicaid recipients. Hospitals are major employers and often a source of considerable community pride.

TABLE 8

STATE SYSTEMS FOR HOSPITAL RATE SETTING
FOR MEDICAID

States with Older Systems	States with Systems Started in 1981, Before 1981 Act	States with Systems Started Since 1981 Act	States with Systems Under Serious Consideration
California (1980)[a]	Florida (July 1)	Alabama[b]	Minnesota
Colorado (1974)	Georgia (January 1)	Illinois	Nebraska
Idaho (1980)	Mississippi (July 1)	Kentucky	Ohio
Maryland (1977)		Missouri	Pennsylvania
Massachusetts (1974)		North Carolina	Washington[c]
Michigan (1976)[a]			
New Jersey (1974)			
New York (1970)			
Rhode Island (1974)			
Wisconsin (1979)			

SOURCE: Personal communications, Health Care Financing Administration, Office of Alternative Reimbursement Systems, May and June 1982.

Note: Some rates are set under experimental authority by HHS waiver, others as "alternative" systems under payments statute.

a. New methodology was implemented in January 1982, after 1981 act.

b. Alabama's system was submitted and approved under the law preceding the 1981 act, then reapproved thereafter.

c. Washington operated an experimental system applicable to some hospitals between 1977 and 1981; it dropped that system and has now applied to HHS for approval for a different methodology, to take effect July 1, 1982.

States may find it more attractive to reduce Medicaid benefits or eligibility than to "take on" the hospital lobby. For all these reasons, state rate setting, while possible, was not popular before 1981.

The 1981 act eliminated altogether the federal requirement for reasonable cost reimbursement. States are now required to pay only the "reasonable and adequate" rates needed to meet the costs of "efficiently and economically operated facilities"—taking into consideration the special needs of institutions serving disproportionate numbers of the poor—and to assure "reasonable access" to services of "adequate quality." As interpreted by federal administrators, this language means that states can set ceilings on next year's payments that are independent of either (1) what any *particular* hospital spends (or wants to spend) or (2) increases in the costs of goods and services used by hospitals—although how far states can go has yet to be established by a definitive court ruling. In addition to the change in legislation, the HCFA approval process has apparently eased considerably, so that states' changes are easier to implement. Thus, the meaning of "rate setting" has changed. In fiscal terms, this is probably the single most important change enacted by the 1981 legislation. The Congressional Budget Office estimated that this provision would reduce federal spending by $250 million even in FY 1982, its first year. Whether these savings are realized will depend on how many and which states make changes, whether the new reimbursement systems withstand lawsuits, and how successful they are in controlling costs.

As a result of these changes and of increased fiscal pressure generally, many states are moving to employ new arrangements or to tighten existing alternative systems. As table 8 showed, five states have established completely new alternative systems since the 1981 act, and California and Illinois have revamped their earlier rate-setting systems. Other states are seriously considering alternative systems, and still others are taking lesser measures to change payment levels. (For example, Vermont has reduced its payments from 100 to 90 percent of Medicare allowable costs.)

The biggest changes have occurred in Illinois, California, and Michigan. The reimbursement change in Illinois is an effort to control overall Medicaid expenditures per hospital as well as rates per day or per procedure. The new system is expected to achieve an estimated $106 million reduction in payments for FY 1982, its first year. The system has worked as follows: First, the state estimated the expected utilization level for each hospital. After hospitals were given an opportunity to revise these estimates, the FY 1979 costs per unit (day or visit) of services for each hospital were updated to project expected spending levels for the hospital during the budget period. (A hospital inflation index developed by Data Resources Inc., a "market basket of inputs" approach, was used to make these projections.) The state then projected its own spending for total hospital services for the budget period by multiplying each hospital's projected unit cost figure by estimated utilization and summing the results across hospitals. After comparing this total with available state funds, the state cut the rates for all hospitals by 14.3 percent— the amount necessary to fit within the Medicaid program's own budget. This apparent ability to tailor payments to the state's ability to pay (if upheld in court) will be a major improvement in control over spending and an enormous departure from past practice and from Medicare-style reasonable cost reimbursement of hospital spending.

There are two available adjustments to ease the impact on hospitals. First, if hospitals cut utilization, their rate can be increased to make up the 14 percent cut. Second, special relief is given to hospitals serving a disproportionately high volume of Medicaid patients. The rates for hospitals serving a population that includes at least 25 percent Medicaid patients are increased on a sliding scale up to the full amount of the 14 percent reduction (although it would take nearly 100 percent Medicaid utilization to get back the full 14 percent). The typical result of this adjustment is somewhat higher rates to hospitals heavily dependent on Medicaid. For FY 1983, further reductions in hospital payments will be made. Hospitals rates are to be increased by 10 percent per unit, but the state plans to limit the number of days it is willing to pay for. Days that exceed the eightieth percentile for length of stay by diagnosis will not be paid for at all.

California sought to limit its rate for FY 1982 for each hospital to 6 percent per discharge above its allowable costs for the previous year. This is the type of system California was forced to abandon under legal challenge in the mid-1970s. Several lawsuits have again been brought against the state, on the ground that a flat 6 percent cap does not satisfy the 1981 act's requirements. A federal district court judge agreed and invalidated the system on June 23, 1982.[12] She held that the Medicaid program had not found that the 6 percent increase would indeed meet the costs of efficiently operated hospitals but in fact had ignored contrary evidence and had simply made the best case it could that the previously set 6 percent legislative limit was valid. The judge held further that the state's assurance of compliance made to HHS therefore "had no reasonable basis," that adopting the cap was "arbitrary and capricious," and that implementing the system without such a finding was "unlawful" and permanently enjoined. If, as seems likely, this ruling is upheld on appeal, California will have to continue paying hospitals under its previous system. Whether the ruling will require the state to make retroactive higher payments to hospitals is still in litigation, and the ultimate fiscal impact is therefore unclear, though it will surely be substantial.

Meanwhile, the California state legislature prepared a different alternative system for paying hospitals, and on June 25 approved a plan for a "special negotiator" in the governor's office[13] beginning July 1st to conclude "selective provider contracts" on rates and other terms directly with (1) individual or groups of private hospitals, (2) county health systems, or (3) competing alternative prepaid health plans (like health maintenance organizations and other organized systems). This Medi-Cal "czar," as the holder of the office is popularly known, is to have maximum discretion to reduce spending through direct negotiation or competitive bids, establishing whatever payment methods are deemed desirable. Beneficiaries will be able to receive services only through the contracting entities. After a year, the czar is meant to operate through the framework of an independent agency. As soon as HHS approval is received (the waiver request was pending as of July 1982), the czar is expected to move first to deal with the most expensive hospitals. A "fall-back" rate-setting system is also being prepared. If approved and fully inplemented, California's new system would be the most significant departure from previous methods of financing and delivering health care services; the negotiation may move beyond hospitals to other services as well.

Michigan reduced its payments under its new prospective payment system by paying on the basis of each hospital's actual per diem costs three years prior to the budget year, projected forward by a hospital cost index. The hospital cost index contains an inflation component (market basket style) and a factor that reflects expected volume changes. Under this system, if a hospital increases its spending faster than the index rises, the hospital will not be reimbursed for the excess spending.

Pennsylvania plans to apply an 8 percent limit on the annual increase in each hospital's daily rates. This approach is similar to that in California and subject to the same judicial attack. Other states would like to follow with percentage increase limits because they are simply to apply, but these states will probably await a more definitive court ruling on the validity of such limits or further changes in federal legislation.

All these approaches have strengths and weaknesses. The California approach of percentage cap per discharge accepts each hospital's current year as the base from which to limit future increases; thus this approach does not address any overspending built in during the more generous "reasonable cost" regime. California's stringent percentage cap would allow strong rate control to be exercised (with almost any limit the state desires). The cap amount also seems likely to be a political matter each year in the legislature, as it was in California this past session, which is likely to continue its vulnerability to legal attack. In addition, the system does not feature total budget control, since the number of admissions may change. In contrast, the systems in Illinois and Michigan do cut into recent spending increases by going back three years for the rate base. However, Illinois is more generous than California in the increases allowed for inflation. Illinois potentially has more budget control than California because of the former's apparent ability to reduce each hospital's rates to keep overall spending within budget. But this tight budget control also makes the Illinois system a likely target for judicial invalidation as unrelated to the costs of efficient hospital operation. Furthermore, neither Illinois's nor California's approach addresses hospital objections that the caps hurt hospitals more if they have been efficient in the past than if they were inefficient and consequently have more "slack" in their rate bases.

Control over hospital rates and overall expenditures by Medicaid programs alone poses series problems, as has already been noted. Control by one payer may not force hospitals to become more efficient; instead it could cause private hospitals to shift their unmet costs to private payers through changes in their charge structure. (This is probably possible only in hospitals where Medicaid patients are a small percentage of all patients.) Hospitals would then be financed relatively more by private insurance premiums and less by federal and state taxes. Alternatively, private hospitals could shift patients, and perhaps even refuse to participate in Medicaid. Public facilities that had a high proportion of Medicaid patients and were unable to shift costs because of a relatively low insured patient population would have to cut back on care (as in staffing) or make other economies (as in capital acquisitions), seek other aid, or close.

States may have to give special rate assistance to hospitals with a large volume of Medicaid patients, as Illinois and California have done, and as is apparently contemplated by the 1981 act. If the states do not mitigate the impact of the rate reduction, there will be no federal matching payments, and deficits of public hospitals will have to be financed entirely by city and county governments.

Nursing Home Payment

States have made fewer recent changes in their nursing home payment systems and payment levels than they have in those for hospitals for two reasons: First, there has been less change in the legal authority of nursing homes under federal standards. As was just noted, the 1981 act authorized, for the first time, significant departures from cost reimbursement for each hospital. In contrast, the 1981 nursing home changes merely modified earlier standards, clarifying the authority of states to undertake rate setting for homes. (The nursing home changes were implemented by regulation in October 1981, along with the 1981 act's changes, but the nursing home statutory provision had actually been changed a year earlier.) Second, most states seem to have been reasonably satisfied with the existing methods and levels of nursing home payment, since they have largely been able to accomplish their fiscal goals already, given their legal authority and economic leverage over homes.

During the 1970s, states were far more active in restricting nursing home payments than in curtailing hospital reimbursement. Medicaid programs have a large stake in nursing home economy measures because nursing home payments typically take the single largest share of a program's budget. In FY 1979, as table 4 showed, nursing homes claimed 42.3 percent of all provider payments—18.4 percent for intermediate care, 16.5 percent for skilled care, and 7.4 percent for intermediate care for the mentally retarded. Economically, there are several reasons why Medicaid programs have been able to control nursing home rates. In contrast to the situation with respect to hospitals, states have enormous leverage with nursing homes because they are by far the dominant payer. Medicaid directly accounts for almost half of the homes' revenues nationwide, and most of the rest comes from presumably cost-conscious individuals rather than from relatively generous insurers. States pay a share of the cost of care for about 60 percent of nursing home patients. When it is necessary for Medicaid to contribute to any patient's care, that person becomes a Medicaid patient. At that time, Medicaid rates determine per diem payments for patients and thus set the cost of care by limiting the available resources of homes and the style of care they can provide. In contrast, the standard costs and operating styles of hospitals are set by more generous insurers—Medicare and private coverage.

Finally, the consequences of holding down payment levels are different for nursing homes and hospitals. If Medicaid pays relatively low rates for hospital care, private hospitals can refuse to accept patients, who can then turn to public hospitals—funded in large measure by state and local governments. When states set Medicaid nursing home rates so low as to dissuade homes from accepting indigent patients, the patients either remain in their communities and go without care, or they remain "backed up" in hospitals—supported partly by Medicaid but largely by Medicare.

Legally, states have long had more flexibility in setting payment rates for nursing homes than for payments to hospitals. In the early years of the Medicaid program, states had great discretion in setting nursing home rates. Many set uniform charges or flat payment ceilings, and the courts supported the authority of states to set rates on the basis of what their budgets could afford rather than on the costs incurred by homes. A major legislative victory for nursing homes occurred in 1972, when Congress mandated that they be paid on a "reasonably cost-related basis" beginning in 1976. Although this provision was slow to be implemented, it surely played a role in the rapid nursing home price increases of the late 1970s.

Although reimbursement rates were thus tied to costs, states were still permitted considerable discretion in setting rates. First, they could choose between prospective and retrospective systems; most states have chosen the former, thought to be more economical because they may encourage homes to live within a budgeted amount. They could then decide whether homes should be grouped by size, ownership, geographic area, and so on; whether total costs or individual cost centers should be limited; whether percentile ceilings should be set on allowable costs (and how high they should set); what kind of inflation allowances should be used in projecting targets in prospective systems or in setting interim rates in retrospective systems; whether efficiency bonuses should be employed; whether specific incentives to encourage higher quality or the admission of patients requiring heavy care should be included; and how capital costs (including profit for investor-owned homes) should be paid for.

All these choices can be made stringently or leniently, so many states have fairly stringent systems while others have more generous arrangements.

There are several reasons why nursing home payments have always received so much more attention from Medicaid authorities than have hospital rates. More money is involved overall, and the rate of increase in spending for nursing homes is greater than for hospitals. Moreover, states have always had more legal flexibility in nursing home payment than they have for hospitals, and controlling the former is technically easier to do. Nursing care is less complex, its individual services tend to be nonacute, and homes are not providers of last resort, so restrictions are more acceptable than in the hospital sector. Furthermore, nursing homes have less political appeal than do hospitals, since nursing homes suffer from an unsavory image of exploiting the elderly and disabled and from periodic outright scandals.[14]

Unlike hospitals, most nursing homes are for-profit operations and less likely to benefit from community charity, pride, and political support. Moreover, the role of publicly run homes is far less vital than that of public hospitals. An exception is ICF/MR, for, as has already been noted, by far most of ICF/MR beds are in public institutions. Significantly, ICF/MR payments are growing faster than any other Medicaid category, as more of these homes are certified to receive Medicaid payment and as prices rise to upgrade participating homes to federal quality standards. But higher Medicaid spending, heavily subsidized by the federal match, may nonetheless save a state money as compared with the cost for a state to fully fund its own facilities at somewhat lower rates.

The 1980 act softened "reasonable-cost related" reimbursement requirements for nursing home payment. Now states are only required to pay rates that are "reasonable and adequate" to meet the necessary costs of "efficiently and economically operated facilities." This language allows greater state control over rate setting and, presumably, over program spending, but less state discretion than had existed before the 1972 federal amendments. This 1980 change is extremely important for another reason as well: It is the standard of payment to which the 1981 act also shifted hospital payment. The 1980 legislation was not implemented until the 1981 amendments were, for FY 1982, beginning on October 1, 1981, but the final regulations increase state discretion even more. Instead of being required to get HCFA approval for changes in method and rates, states are now merely required to submit assurances of compliance with the statute and to renew them every year the rates are in effect.

State payments for nursing homes have changed less than have those for hospitals since their respective federal requirements were changed. In part this situation reflects slow implementation of nursing home regulations at the federal level, as was just mentioned. (In contrast, federal hospital payment regulations under the 1981 act were in place by October 1981.) More important, previous nursing home provisions permitted states a greater initial degree of control over rates. States such as California and Illinois had applied ceilings to individual facilities at the fiftieth percentile of industry costs, had employed inflation factors which limited payment increases, and had generally achieved some control over growth rates in each home's payments. Nonetheless several states did alter payment policies after the 1980 law. Connecticut, Georgia, Kentucky, Michigan, Nevada, Rhode Island, Virginia and Washington reported limiting rates by reducing profit factors, limiting or changing inflation allowances, changing treatment of sales, or reducing ceilings on total costs or particular cost centers.

Flat-rate payment may be an even stronger cost-containing approach. It deviates the most dramatically from "reasonably cost related" approaches and has the potential for greater savings but can be more or less generous depending upon the method used. Arkansas, for example, has changed its system to pay a flat rate set at the eightieth percentile of expected costs for each of six classes of homes. Expected costs are projected using an inflation factor determined by the state. It is not clear that this method will reduce rates. Oklahoma's new system is similar but will cease to use percentile limits after 1981, paying full historical costs plus inflation increases. Utah has also introduced a flat-rate system, but its flat rates are negotiated with the industry, and rates are said to have increased markedly.

States have also made changes that increase costs. Illinois has changed its method of determining its patient-related nursing cost reimbursement, and the state expects the new system to cost more. Florida has also adopted a new reimbursement system in which rates are tied to patient condition, and this state, too, expects its outlays to increase. Maryland is considering adopting a similar arrangement.

Clearly there is a tension between economizing and providing sufficient support for adequate care, and states have had longer to seek out the appropriate balance for nursing homes than for hospitals. The recent relative lack of nursing home rate-setting activity probably reflects the great deal of attention given the matter in the past. Many states may be satisfied with their methods of payment. In many states further constraints on nursing home rates are likely to affect the quality of care they provide and the access of Medicaid recipients to beds. Reductions in quality may be politically unacceptable, while reduction in access may be fiscally undesirable because patients remain in hospitals awaiting placement. The full effects of payment policy on cost control, quality, and access are not well understood, so that states may be wary of taking drastic actions.

Physician Payment

The discretion that states have over Medicaid payment to physicians has always been even broader than the discretion states have over nursing home payment, and Medicaid programs have traditionally paid physicians less than does Medicare or private insurers. In contrast to the Medicaid statute, the Medicare statute mandated a relatively generous form of payment that paid almost all physicians the fees they usually charged their patients in the previous year. This system pays "usual, customary, and reasonable" fees and is thus called the UCR payment system. The Medicaid statute, however, has never imposed any particular method of physician payment on state programs. Only two major requirements for Medicaid payments were traditionally imposed: that they be high enough to assure reasonable access to care for beneficiaries yet that they not exceed Medicare levels.

Most states initially opted to pay Medicare fees or at least to use UCR payment principles, preferred by physicians because levels change with physicians' fees. The main reasons were probably the attraction of being administratively consistent with Medicare, the other major public payer, and the desire to achieve high participation by physicians and thus relatively good access to care for Medicaid beneficiaries. By the mid-1970s Medicare itself began to limit UCR payment levels (called "CPR"—for customary, prevailing, and reasonable—under Medicare). In brief, the annual growth rate of fees above a certain high percentile is limited to the level of an exogenously determined inflation factor. The general result has been that physicians have found that their UCR fees for an increasing number

of procedures have reached the allowable ceiling and now can grow
only at the approved rate. (The actual system is quite complex.)

Several Medicaid programs have imposed even stronger limits
and ceilings on the UCR system. Over time, more programs have
changed to fee schedules (which are more straightforward than the
UCR system, which pays each doctor individually)—either by applying such low UCR ceilings that essentially all fees are at the
ceiling, or by creating a uniform schedule based on relative value
scales listing each procedure or on some other basis.

In general, when Medicaid cuts must be made, programs very
often turn to further restrictions on physician fees. In 1975, for
example, Massachusetts slashed fees 30 percent across the board,
and it has raised fees only slightly since then. New York held physician fees at 1969 levels throughout the 1970s, with only a brief
interlude of slightly higher payment. Many states maintain the
appearance of UCR payment (preferred by physicians) while drastically altering its substance. This can be done by postponing "up-
dates" of physician fee "profiles" (the pattern of past charges used
to compute payments); thus, for example, 1981 payment may still
be based on 1978 profiles, which are themselves based on 1977 fees.
Alternatively, Medicaid programs may be more selective about fee
restrictions. When Michigan cut most fees by 10 percent in FY 1981,
for example, fees for primary physicians' services—the most basic
care—were left unchanged. The idea was that specialists' procedures
were overcompensated relative to generalists' procedures and that
maintaining primary fees would help maintain access to basic care.

Over time, some states have regularly increased fees, either by
maintaining Medicaid payment rates at Michigan levels (which are
updated annually) or in other ways. But most states have somehow
restricted physician payments. There is evidence that states which
are more generous in eligibility or service coverage are less generous
in physician payment.[15] Also, states using fee schedules pay lower
rates than do states that use the UCR system of payment. The ratio
of Medicaid to Medicare fees for specialists is shown in table 9 by
state. The correlation of high ratios with UCR (Medicare-style) payment is remarkable: Fee schedule states are almost exclusively low-
paying states. While in several states Medicaid pays the same as
Medicare and in three states Medicaid pays more,[16] in most states,
Medicaid pays substantially less. Moreover, almost all the large
Medicaid programs have quite low fees by Medicare standards. The
biggest Medicaid programs are all in the bottom half; California,

TABLE 9

MEDICAID-TO-MEDICARE FEE
RATIOS, FOR SPECIALISTS,
FY 1980

Rank	State	Medical Payment Method[a]	Ratio
1	Nevada	FS	1.13
2	Minnesota	UCR	1.02
3	South Carolina	UCR	1.02
4	Alaska	UCR	1.00
5	Indiana	UCR	1.00
6	Iowa	UCR	1.00
7	Nebraska	UCR	1.00
8	North Carolina	UCR	1.00
9	Oklahoma	UCR	1.00
10	Texas	UCR	1.00
11	Utah	UCR	1.00
12	Wisconsin	UCR	1.00
13	Wyoming	UCR	1.00
14	Kentucky	UCR	0.99
15	Delaware	UCR	0.99
16	North Dakota	UCR	0.98
17	Louisiana	UCR	0.98
18	New Mexico	UCR	0.94
19	Arkansas	UCR	0.92
20	Hawaii	UCR	0.90
21	Tennessee	UCR	0.90
22	South Dakota	UCR	0.88
23	Idaho	FS	0.85
24	Oregon	FS	0.83
25	Michigan	FS	0.79
26	Georgia	UCR	0.77
27	Kansas	UCR	0.76
28	Washington	FS	0.73
29	Montana	FS	0.72
30	New Hampshire	FS	0.68
31	Vermont	FS	0.68
32	Mississippi	FS	0.65
33	Virginia	FS	0.65
34	West Virginia	FS	0.65
35	Ohio	UCR	0.61
36	Maine	FS	0.61
37	Illinois	FS	0.61
38	Alabama	UCR	0.60
39	District of Columbia	FS	0.59
40	Missouri	FS	0.57
41	Massachusetts	FS	0.56

TABLE 9 (continued)

Rank	State	Medical Payment Method[a]	Ratio
42	California	FS	0.54
43	Colorado	FS	0.51
44	Connecticut	FS	0.48
45	Rhode Island	FS	0.44
46	Florida	FS	0.44
47	New Jersey	FS	0.43
48	Maryland	FS	0.43
49	Pennsylvania	FS	0.29
50	New York	FS	0.24

SOURCE: John Holahan, "Paying for Physician Services in State Medicaid Programs," Urban Institute Working Paper No. 2015–01, July 1982.

a. FS is fee schedule, and UCR is usual, customary, and reasonable fees (Medicare style).

Massachusetts, New York, and Pennsylvania are all very low indeed. New York's program was lowest, paying specialists in 1980 at rates which were 24 percent of Medicare levels.

Overall, Medicaid programs have succeeded in restricting growth in physician fees. As table 4 showed, physician payments grew (relatively) very slowly between 1975 and 1979—only 7.0 percent per year, about half the average growth rate for total Medicaid spending.

To a great extent, however, such "success" is probably pennywise and pound-foolish. Physician fees claim a very small—and declining—share of Medicaid spending: only 10.2 percent in 1975 and 8.0 percent in 1979. In contrast, during those years physicians received 21.4 percent and 21.5 percent of total national personal health care spending; total spending on their services rose at an annual rate of 13.0 percent.[17] Physicians have clearly been squeezed hard by Medicaid. This "success" in paying relatively less for physicians' services clearly has its cost in reducing the willingness of physicians to serve Medicaid patients—all the more so since, under Medicaid, providers may not charge supplementary fees to recipients themselves as they may under Medicare and almost all private plans. Measuring physician participation in Medicaid is difficult, but it seems absolutely clear that reducing fees reduces participation.[18]

Holding down physician fees may also be pound-foolish because reduced physician participation seems to drive many beneficiaries to substitute other services at greater cost to Medicaid: hospital emergency rooms and outpatient departments, even inpatient services. As table 4 showed, while physician payments have stagnated, payments for outpatient hospital care have climbed rapidly—some 22.0 percent per year between 1975 and 1979. Not all this change is due to Medicaid program policy, since hospital outpatient use has been growing among the general population as well. Preliminary results from other Urban Institute research, however, tend to show that *raising* Medicaid physician fees might well actually *reduce* hospital inpatient spending per beneficiary and overall Medicaid spending.[19] It would seem that enlightened Medicaid policy should seek to reduce expensive reliance on hospitals, even at the cost of some increase in physician payments.

It is not clear why Medicaid programs have worked so much harder to limit physician fees than to curb hospital costs when the latter are not only far larger but also growing much faster. The simplest explanation is that when Medicaid programs are under severe fiscal pressure to *do something*, physician fee controls are attractive. Not only does everyone "know" that physicians in general earn "too much," whereas most hospitals are "nonprofit," but Medicaid-dependent physicians are often a low-status subcategory of physicians, often derided even by fellow professionals for running "Medicaid mills" of high volume and low quality.

Moreover, action on physician fees is easily taken; slowing their growth and even freezing them has long been possible under federal law. Hospital controls, in contrast, cannot be so drastic and are much more difficult to implement, even after the 1981 changes in federal law and regulations. Also, Medicaid physicians are typically less powerful politically than are hospitals. Whereas hospitals usually enjoy considerable general community support (and employ a considerable number of local residents), physicians who earn a significant share of their income from Medicaid typically do not. There are also relatively few hospitals compared with the number of physicians, so that the former may speak with a more unified and potent political voice.

The only change made by the 1981 reconciliation act in physician reimbursement was a technical amendment to remove Medicare levels as an upper limit on Medicaid fees. Lawmakers feared that the previous law might have inhibited some states from using statewide fee schedules. Because Medicare permits such wide variations in fees, use of statewide fee schedules might have resulted in fees for some physicians that exceeded their Medicare levels. The prevalence of fee schedules among states shows that this was not a large problem. At any rate, under the new statute, states are completely free to establish fee schedules without worrying about Medicare payment levels.

This 1981 act prompted little change in states' physician payment policies as one might suspect, given the small changes made in federal law. No state reported changing from a UCR system to a fee schedule for FY 1982. States with UCR systems reported annual fee increases as usual. One exception is South Carolina, which lowered its UCR ceiling from 100 percent of Medicare-allowable charges to 90 percent. Many states with fee schedules—including Connecticut, Illinois, Maryland, Michigan, and New York—did not increase their rates (again, common practice in difficult years). California, Georgia, and Pennsylvania increased Medicaid fees but by less than private fees increased. Oregon reduced its Medicaid fees for surgery, anesthesiology, and certain office procedures.

One development of interest is an attempt by some states to provide incentives to encourage physicians to deliver services outside hospitals. For example, Colorado is exploring a payment system that would share with physicians any savings from reduced hospitalization. Washington increased fees for primary care services relative to more specialized (often in-hospital) care. Missouri is considering increasing fees for evening office visits and for deliveries performed in the office. Kansas increased its fees for 137 surgical and diagnostic procedures if they are performed out of the hospital.

Other Developments

A related development with regard to payment practices is an unusual provision of the 1981 act. The secretary of the Department of Health and Human Services is empowered to give states waivers to restrict the freedom of choice for beneficiaries by limiting them to providers who meet state standards for "efficient and economic provision of covered care." This language seems to allow states to exclude what they consider unduly high-charging providers from payment altogether. As of May 1982, we had learned of no state that planned for such far-reaching changes. One unfortunate circumstance for Medicaid programs is that they must often rely disproportionately for services to the poor on institutions which are among the most expensive providers—public and teaching hospitals, especially those in large cities. Over time, states may show more interest in the possibility of channeling more beneficiaries to particular providers in exchange for more control over spending, short of health maintenance organizations (which are considered in the next section). As of July 1982, California planned to have its "czar" arrange exclusive contracts with some inpatient providers, as has already been noted.

Although this report cannot cover all cost-containment strategies in detail, two others deserve quick mention. Hospital outpatient (and most clinic) rates are subject to direct Medicaid controls, and recent federal and state attention has been directed to bringing rates into line with private physician office visits. Also, since the 1981 act, drug and equipment suppliers can be paid on the basis of competitive bidding rather than on the basis of their own costs.

Other Measures

States may take a variety of other measures to reduce expenditures. Significant ones fall into three broad areas: (1) administration, (2) new delivery arrangements, and (3) alternatives to nursing home care. States have had strong incentives to improve administration in the past and now have new flexibility to explore the latter two areas.

Administration

States have been given added reason to improve administration by the 1981 act: One percentage point of the 3 percent reduction in federal matching payment is forgiven if the state can prove it saved at least that amount through reduction of fraud and abuse (or at least in FY 1982) by third-party recoveries. For several years states have attempted to increase revenues from third parties other than their own Medicaid programs. One is the Medicare program for aged or disabled Medicaid eligibles; other potentially available third-party resources include private insurance, the Veterans' Administration, the Black Lung Program, and the Civilian Health and Medicaid Program of the Uniformed Services (CHAMPU—largely military dependents). Such efforts have their limits, however. Many Medicaid beneficiaries cannot afford private insurance; moreover, most private insurance contracts specifically exclude care for which government program payment is available, although states may by statute invalidate such provisions.

Administrative efficiencies of other types are also often sought. For Medicaid, unlike other state agencies, efficiency does not normally mean doing state business with fewer or lower-cost employees. Rather, it means saving money on the provider payments and other outside expenses that constitute 95 percent of Medicaid spending. Probably the most important step here is improving eligibility determinations and verifications to assure that payments are not made for ineligible beneficiaries. Despite federal penalties for high error rates and federal encouragement for better employee training, many states have lagged in this area. By the latter half of the 1970s, however, many programs had embarked on major eligibility efforts, retraining eligibility workers, issuing photo-identification cards of eligibles, and the like.

Even more important, by 1980 almost all states had finally complied with federal requirements to automate their eligibility systems, as part of the Medicaid Management Information System (MMIS). MMIS allows rapid understanding and response to many particular problems—and not just for eligibility determinations. Avoiding duplicate payments to providers, deciding on and implementing particular utilization controls through claims processing, assuring that the correct amount is paid (e.g., paying for a service at the rate in effect when it was provided, not at the later and probably higher rate at time of payment)—all these tasks virtually require automated processing.

Other administrative efforts include better auditing of Medicaid intermediaries (if the state does not pay bills itself), going to competitive bidding for choice of intermediary, and even taking over direct payment of bills by the state.

Alternative Delivery Arrangements

Changing provider arrangements from cost-based, fee-for-service care is a major reform that has been little implemented by state Medicaid programs. Some efforts, however, have been made. The major alternative is the health maintenance organization (HMO). HMOs are medical organizations which usually have their own doctors and hospitals and which contract to deliver all needed services for a fixed, advance payment per enrollee. Their fixed-budget incentive and increased control over medical resource allocation are thought to make them less expensive per enrollee than the fee-for-service system otherwise used by Medicaid. Just how large the savings can be, however, is debatable, as is the manner any savings are achieved.[20] (There is concern that lower costs come from attracting low users of care rather than from more efficient provision of care.) It should also be noted that HMOs do not provide long-term nursing home care, which makes up a large fraction of Medicaid spending. HMOs are the principal but not the only means of altering provider structure and incentives away from cost-based, fee-for-service delivery.

HMOs, which have historically accounted for only a tiny fraction of Medicaid spending, are limited to only a few states, chiefly California and Michigan. There have been many impediments to the growth of HMO contracting by Medicaid programs, the most important of which is that there are no HMOs available in most of the country. Other problems are these: (1) Federal Medicaid regulations have been oriented to cost and charge reimbursement per service and have long hindered advance capitation payments to HMOs, which might then "profit" from economizing. Setting appropriate HMO capitation rates for different kinds of patients is also difficult. Failure to set appropriate rates can lead to the "creaming" of low users or to the acquisition of too easy profits, or both. (2) Medicaid eligibility is an on-again, off-again phenomenon; there is far less stability in welfare rolls and among the medically needy than there is among the employed populations with which HMOs customarily deal. This instability not only might disrupt HMOs' cash flow but could also interfere with HMOs' ability to manage spending and to economize. (3) HMOs have incentives to underserve patients just as fee-for-service providers are motivated to overserve. Problems with maintaining quality were a major factor in the ill-fated proliferation of Medi-Cal HMOs in California in the early 1970s. (4) Because most Medicaid eligibles have no premium payment or cost-sharing obligations under conventional coverage, these people often have very little reason to join an HMO as an alternative. Thus, unless an HMO can offer cash rebates, longer eligibility, or some other inducement to Medicaid enrollees, getting them to join HMOs might require the Medicaid program to restrict the free choice of provider by eligibles.

Other prepaid arrangements are also being developed. They typically involve placing individual private physicians at risk for overspending or providing some other incentive for physicians to monitor the provision of services to patients. One innovation is not to prepay for all care for a person but simply to put one primary care physician in charge of guiding and monitoring all care provided to a beneficiary (with varying degrees of fiscal incentive). In the private sector, Safeco in the West and Group Health of Northeast Ohio have used this approach. Doctors are paid on a capitation basis for each enrollee's physician visits, hospital outpatient care, and office-based laboratory and radiological procedures. Any profit or loss in providing such services is borne by the physician. A second insurance fund covers inpatient care, referrals to specialist physicians, prescriptions, and other tests and x-rays. The primary physician must authorize all referrals, hospital admissions, and the like, and that physician shares in some of the risk of overspending by that fund.

Special waivers from HHS traditionally were required to permit nontraditional payment mechanisms or limitation of Medicaid patients' right to receive care from any provider. But several provisions in the 1981 act attempted to increase the states' use of prepayment arrangements. With regard to HMOs, the former 50 percent ceiling on public program participation in each HMO was increased to 75 percent of total enrollment (even the 75 percent could be exceeded with a waiver). In addition, states were permitted to guarantee HMOs that Medicaid enrollees would retain eligibility for a minimum period of up to six months, with federal matching payments, even if the enrollees would otherwise have lost eligibility. With respect to other new delivery arrangements, such as case management or primary care networks, the 1981 act made waivers of the "freedom of choice" requirement easier for states to get. States may thus limit enrollees' choice of physician under alternative delivery methods. Counties or other units of government also are permitted to act as brokers for Medicaid recipients to give them a choice among several competing alternatives—conventional Medicaid coverage, HMOs, private insurance—again, by liberalized waiver provisions. Moreover, both HMOs and other prepaid arrangements, such as primary care networks, were permitted to provide additional services as a way to attract eligibles. Thus the new legislation dealt with several problems that had been inhibiting delivery system reform: making it easier for programs to contract with HMOs, broadening the kinds of delivery arrangements which could be used by the program, and creating incentives for recipients to join alternatives. Problems such as setting appropriate capitation rates for acute-care services remain for the states to resolve—as does the vexing problem of long-term care, not addressed by these alternatives.

The response to the legislative efforts to encourage new delivery arrangements has been mixed. Some states—for example, Georgia,

Hawaii, and Ohio—are reported to be considering initiating or expanding use of HMOs. Colorado received a freedom-of-choice waiver to require Medicaid recipients in one county to receive services from a designated HMO. Several states, however, informed us that significant expansion was unlikely because they had so few HMOs.

A few states have applied for freedom-of-choice waivers to develop case management or primary care network arrangements. Probably the most ambitious prepayment scheme is that now being proposed by Massachusetts as a complete replacement for its current Medicaid program. The proposed system's details are not yet entirely fleshed out, but the essential idea is to prepay private intermediaries (which could be provider groups) to assume all responsibility for serving the Medicaid population in exchange for fixed prepayments and an end to almost all Medicaid controls and restrictions. The intermediaries would subcontract with case managers—primary care physicians reimbursed on a fee-for-service basis who must authorize all services—and with HMOs.

Michigan has received a waiver to introduce a program in Wayne County (Detroit) under which 223,000 Medicaid recipients will be given a choice of enrolling in an HMO or enrolling with a private physician known as the primary physician sponsor. The sponsor will receive a payment of three dollars per month for providing case management services expected to reduce the use of hospitals. The state expects that 60,000 more persons will choose to join an HMO and expects savings both from HMOs and from case management.

Maryland is considering a plan that would increase fees to private physicians in return for case management services, would increase payments to neighborhood health centers to encourage them to treat more Medicaid patients, and would develop capitation arrangements with two large Baltimore hospitals. California's Medicaid "czar" is empowered to make numerous prepayment (and other) arrangements for service delivery. Moreover, California is planning to place counties partially at risk for the provision of services to the "medically indigent" (a state-only category of eligibles). The counties could in turn provide services directly or could develop prepayment or other arrangements with private providers.

In general, states appear to be approaching the new freedom of choice authority with caution. Since relatively few HMOs and even fewer primary care networks or case management arrangements are in place, developing them will take time. Moreover, Medicaid programs must be willing to pay them enough to make it worth their while to assume new populations, particularly where they must assume financial risks. New providers may logically seek the protection of an extra "risk premium" for dealing with an unfamiliar and needy Medicaid population. Yet, the Medicaid programs' ability to pay is, if anything, limited to below-normal rates. After all, they have typically paid less than going rates to conventional physicians and are now beginning to pay lower rates to hospitals as well. It could prove quite difficult to promote alternative arrangements and reduce overall expenditures at the same time. In this sense, many prepayment options may constitute long-term rather than intermediate economizing options.

Alternatives to Nursing Homes

Interest in providing alternatives to long term institutional care has been increasing. Many observers have long argued that Medicaid has a distinct institutional bias and that many people who are now being served in nursing homes could be served better and at lower cost with community-based care. Prior to the 1981 act, Medicaid programs could cover home health and personal care services if prescribed by a physician and supervised by a nurse. It was argued, however, that the "medical necessity" required to cover community care deterred states from offering appropritate homemaker and other nonmedical services that might be necessary to keep people out of nursing homes. The essential problem is that Medicaid operates on a medical insurance model, while long-term care is in large measure a matter of social and custodial as well as medical services.

Under the new legislation, states may apply for waivers to cover home and community-based services for persons who otherwise would require care in a skilled nursing or intermediate care facility. States must assure HHS that patients will be carefully evaluated with respect to their need for SNF/ICF care, that patients in need will be given a choice of nursing home or community care, and that per capita spending under the waiver does not exceed what spending would have been without it. Waivers are to be granted for three years and can be extended for an additional three. With a waiver, states may provide case management; homemaker, home health aide, and personal care services; adult day care, respite care, and similar services.

The regulations implementing the statute attempt to impose tight control on the net cost of the new community services. Evidence suggests that community services are likely to increase program costs because they do not really substitute for nursing home care but rather serve a somewhat different, less impaired, and larger noninstitutionalized population.[21] With these concerns in mind, HHS required state assurances that aggregate program costs would not be higher with the community care waiver than without it. How successful the HHS controls will be is problematic. The main problem appears to be that assurances about expected costs either with or without the waiver of necessity rest on estimates. States can, if they choose, manipulate the waiver process by making a rational but high estimate of what costs would have been without the waiver, despite HHS attempts to specify the formula for estimation. Estimates can, legitimately, vary quite widely, since they cannot be made simply by extrapolating from demographic data. Long-term-care costs can be and have been controlled through certificate-of-need policies, preadmission screening, reimbursements rates, benefit limits, and the like. As a result, predicting utilization and costs for new community services is also difficult, and defensible estimates can vary widely. States may want to provide home or community-based services in Medicaid not merely for nursing home care but also in part to reinstate noninstitutional services cut back under other grant programs (especially Title XX social services), or simply to provide better services to people. The possibility of inter-title transfers and Medicaid cost expansion is clear, and it would seem that states could accomplish such expansions through the waiver process if they submit appropriate estimates. Whether budget-conscious reviewers at HHS will disallow waiver requests they find suspicious remains to be seen, and how the Reagan administration will react if actual spending exceeds estimates is not known.

By the summer of 1982, twenty-two states had applied for "community care waivers," seven states had been approved, and many more were planning to apply. The states with approved waiver applications are Florida, Iowa, Kansas, Louisiana, Missouri, Montana and Oregon. California and Tennessee have had applications denied; other are pending. Several waiver applications are intended to provide services to the mentally retarded who otherwise might be in institutions. Others are aimed at both the mentally retarded and the aged and chronically ill.

The home and community-care amendment is a very important part of the 1981 act package. While intended to permit states to reduce Medicaid's bias toward institutionalization of the aged, disabled, mentally ill, and mentally retarded at no increased cost to the states or the federal government, the amendment clearly might repeat the history of other benefits expansions in Medicaid. If it does, federal costs will increase as states conserve on their own spending by shifting into Medicaid services that could otherwise be financed through other federal programs (with less matching funds) or entirely through state dollars.

CHAPTER 4

CONCLUSION

This report has examined the changes in Medicaid policy and practice brought about by the Reagan administration and the 1981 Omnibus Budget Reconciliation Act. The legislation reduced the federal share of Medicaid spending while it increased the options available to states to economize in administering their programs. However, Congress stopped far short of the administration's plan to convert Medicaid into something very like a "block grant" of a fixed dollar amount to states.

The administration proposed a fixed 5 percent "cap" on growth in Medicaid spending, which could otherwise be expected to continue rising between 15 and 20 percent a year. The proposed cap would have put the states under enormous fiscal pressure at the same time that the rest of the administration's proposal would have given the states enormous discretion to reduce and restructure their Medicaid programs. The legislation that was enacted, however, maintained the open-ended federal matching contribution (at a 3 percent lower rate) and the basic free-choice-of-provider, entitlement nature of the program, thus creating far less fiscal pressure on the states and encouraging them to continue past coverage so as to maintain a high federal contribution to the costs of providing indigent medical care.

The fiscal condition of states and their attitudes about Medicaid spending vary widely, and these conditions and attitudes rather than federal policy seem to have been the driving forces behind most recent Medicaid program changes. In fact, the marginal reduction in the federal Medicaid share has played a much less influential role in actions by states than have more general state fiscal problems stemming from the deepening recession and other limits on state revenues.

We have reviewed the choices available to states before and after the 1981 act; the legal, political, and fiscal constraints on choice; and the decisions states have made in the new environment. The main conclusion is that, while states have made important programmatic reductions, wholesale cuts are rather rare. This situation reflects the continuing desire of the states to maintain an open-ended federal contribution to cover certain low-income people or particular medical services that would otherwise be provided wholly at state or local expense. Major Medicaid contractions could increase costs for many states, not reduce them.

Historically, states have attempted to control Medicaid costs through some limits on eligibility (principally by controlling welfare payment standards or by limiting coverage of state-only populations), through limits on the scope of benefits (e.g., the number of physicians visits, hospitals days), through controls on provider payment levels (notably physician fees and nursing home rates but occasionally also hospital rates), and through a number of administrative efforts.

In FY 1982, federally mandated reductions in AFDC eligibility automatically cut Medicaid costs; state freezes in welfare payment standards also cut Medicaid costs. In general, however, states have not made drastic cuts in eligibility, such as eliminating the non-institutionalized medically needy program, because doing so would probably have increased the charity care provided by local public hospitals. Hence, the ultimate effect would have been merely to shift costs to local governments or to private taxpayers. (California is an important exception, however, for that state is planning to shift to counties much of the burden of covering its "medically indigent" people who are not eligible for federal support.) States also try to avoid cutbacks among the institutionalized medically needy, many of whom are elderly, because of the likely adverse political consequences of targeting this highly vulnerable and popularly supported group.

Similarly, states have not eliminated coverage of major optional services. For example, to reduce reliance on more expensive skilled nursing homes, states have chosen to cover intermediate care facilities and state-financed facilities that provide less skilled nursing and personal care. Similarly, states have upgraded facilities caring for the mentally retarded (mainly state operated) to meet Medicaid certification standards and thereby receive federal matching funds for persons eligible for Medicaid. These two optional services have been among the fastest-growing items in Medicaid. They are not likely targets for cuts because states would then bear all the costs for most of these people. State costs would almost surely increase even if total Medicaid costs fell.

State have, however, traditionally imposed limits on drugs and on minor optional services, sometimes even dropping coverage, if only during a temporary budget crunch. Limits on drug coverage include restricting the number and kinds of drugs covered, eliminating over-the-counter drugs, requiring use of generic drugs, and imposing copayments on prescriptions. Several states have eliminated or placed limits on smaller optional services—care by dentists, chiropractors, podiatrists, optometrists, and so on; many states have imposed copayments or limited coverage to certain beneficiaries. As with major services, a major constraint on cutbacks is concern that eliminating one service will simply lead to use of more expensive substitutes.

States have continued previous policies of tight controls on physician fees, despite growing evidence that such constraints lead to increased reliance on hospital outpatient departments and perhaps even to increases in overall spending. But most states have not recently reduced or frozen nursing home rates, mainly because the states had already established control over rate increases in recent years. Further tightening of controls could severely reduce access and quality of care in many states.

In the very important matter of hospital payment, however, FY 1982 represents a significant break from the past. The 1981 legislation greatly reduced federal requirements that had led states to pay each hospital's actual costs. Under the new law and HHS policy, states can set prospective rates below the actual spending by individual hospitals so long as the costs of an efficient operation are met, reasonable access is maintained, and special needs of hospitals that serve disproportionate numbers of poor people are recognized. The practical result of the new payment regime seems to be that states can employ much more stringent payment limits than before, independent of apparent increases in prices hospitals pay to their own employees and suppliers, as well as of attempts by hospitals to increase their rate bases for future years. The exact limit of new state authority, however, must await a definitive court ruling; California's arbitrary 6 percent cap seems to have gone too far, according to one federal District Court. By mid-1982, eighteen states had alternative systems and another eighteen states reported either making or seriously considering payment changes since passage of the 1981 law. In addition, several states have introduced (or reduced) limits on the number of hospital days they will cover, and some are eliminating weekend admissions, reducing coverage of preoperative days, and ending payment for inpatient surgery for services that can be performed on an outpatient basis. In short, Medicaid programs are trying harder than ever before to control hospital costs, which account for almost a third of all spending.

Other effects of the 1981 act will be felt more slowly. While Congress was cutting a multitude of health programs in 1981, it authorized waivers from several Medicaid requirements to allow one important expansion of Medicaid: to provide long term care *outside* nursing homes. Experience suggests that such benefits may increase, not reduce public expenses, since services are costly and programs usually end up serving many more people than would otherwise have entered nursing homes. Federal regulations try to prevent this effect by requiring assurances from states that a state's Medicaid costs with a waiver will not exceed what they would have been without one, but it is not clear the regulations will succeed. Assurances can only be based on estimates, and there is considerable room for manipulation within the bounds of legitimate prediction. For many states, the new provision offers an opportunity to shift the costs of services they now fund (or would like to fund) at full or considerable state expense to the Medicaid program, with its relatively generous, open-ended federal matching funds. By sharing expenses with the federal government, states can get a bargain even if service and spending expand. States may also introduce new services in response to growing demand or in the belief these services will cost less than nursing home care.

By the summer of 1982, twenty-two states had applied for "community-care waivers," and seven had received approvals. The cost of these programs is very likely to increase and the result may be cuts in this or other Medicaid benefits over the long term. But for a time, the new program may well expand services to the elderly and the physically and mentally disabled.

The 1981 law also gave states greater flexibility to promote efficient alternatives to conventional fee-for-service practice—including health maintenance organizations and less structured "case management" and "capitation networks." "Case management" involves paying fees to physicians to manage a patient's total care, while "capitation networks" are prepayment arrangements with primary care physicians. Because such plans are largely untried and face significant implementation problems, states are approaching these mechanisms with caution. With fees already low, it may prove very difficult to attract physicians to new systems and to reward innovation and efficiency without risking increased costs.

States have continued to be very inventive in controlling Medicaid spending, in most respects performing well compared with Medicare or with private insurers. The 1981 act has acted as a modest fiscal spur and as considerable relief from previous federal impediments to new approaches.

While states are constraining the scope of their programs, there are clear limits on their willingness to do so. The major problem is that the poor and chronically ill are in need of some level of medical care and are unable to pay for it. Government support, whether federal, state, or local, is required. With Medicaid states can provide more service to the poor at lower cost to themselves because federal funds match state payments. Thus, maintaining some basic structure of Medicaid eligibility and benefits remains attractive to states, despite the federal cutbacks.

NOTES

NOTES TO INTRODUCTION AND SUMMARY

1. This monograph is part of a series in The Urban Institute's analysis of changing domestic priorities under the Reagan administration, as noted in the Foreword. (For a comprehensive report on the first eighteen months, see John L. Palmer and Isabel V. Sawhill, eds., *The Reagan Experiment* (Washington, D.C.: The Urban Institute Press, 1982).) The series has been funded by a consortium of private foundations and corporations, but the authors' opinions should not, of course, be construed to be those of the Institute or its sponsors.

2. This report is based primarily on the sources listed in this note. (Henceforth we will normally use notes only when specific information comes from other sources.) Official data came from Donald N. Muse and Darwin Sawyer, *The Medicare and Medicaid Data Book, 1981* (Department of Health and Human Services, Health Care Financing Administration, Office of Research and Development: Health Care Financing Program Statistics, HCFA Pub. No. 03128, April 1982). This reference reports data for fiscal years 1973-1979. Earlier years were compiled on a calendar-year basis. See Medicare/Medicaid Management Institute, *Data on the Medicaid Program: Eligibility, Services, Expenditures (United States Department of Health, Education and Welfare, Health Care Financing Administration 1979)* Recent fiscal year data are also available in the *Medicaid State Tables* for each year. Notable examples of past Urban Institute work include a four-part study of Medicaid program responses to the 1974-1975 recession and a study of state fiscal restraints and health policy since 1975. See, e.g., John Holahan, William Scanlon, and Bruce Spitz, *Restructuring Federal Medicaid Controls and Incentives*, Urban Institute paper, June 1977; and Randall R. Bovbjerg, "State and Local Health Policy in an Era of Fiscal Limitations," Urban Institute Working Paper No. 1389-021, August 1981.

The main fifty-state surveys we have used are Lawrence Bartlett and Claudia Hanson, eds., "A Catalog of State Medicaid Program Changes" (Washington, D.C.: State Medicaid Program Information Center, National Governors Association, March 1982) and Intergovernmental Health Policy Project, *Recent or Proposed Changes in State Medicaid Programs* (George Washington University, International Health Policy Project, May 1981, updated edition October 1981). Specifically for this study, John Holahan surveyed ten state Medicaid programs (including all the largest ones) by telephone during March and April 1982. See John Holahan, "1982 Medicaid Program Adjustments: A View From Ten States" Urban Institute Working Paper No. 3076-04, May 1982. The states were California, Connecticut, Florida, Illinois, Kentucky, Maryland, Michigan, New York, Oregon, and Pennsylvania. We also drew upon less systematic recent contacts with Medicaid administrators and observers made in connection with miscellaneous other Urban Institute projects.

A good source on the provisions of the 1981 act, its legislative history, its implementing regulations, and other information is the Commerce Clearing House, *Medicare and Medicaid Guide*, especially paragraphs 24,000 ff. (Chicago, looseleaf service, updated biweekly).

NOTES TO CHAPTER 1

1. The District of Columbia and four territories also participate; for convenience, however, all jurisdictions will be referred to indiscriminately as "states."

2. Since 1975 by federal statute, Guam, Puerto Rico, and the Virgin Islands have been exempt from this "free choice of provider" requirement. See Commerce Clearing House, *Medicare and Medicaid Guide* para. 14,525.

3. Again, Guam, Puerto Rico, and the Virgin Islands are different, being subject to fixed dollar limits.

4. Congressional Budget Office estimate of January 1982 (not counting any program changes in 1982 and assuming an average federal share of 54 percent).

5. See Linda E. Demkovich, "For States Squeezed by Medicaid Costs, The Worst Crunch Is Yet to Come, *National Journal,* January 10, 1981, pp. 44-49; and Mark S. Freeland and Carol Ellen Schendler, "National Health Expenditures: Short-Term Outlook and Long-Term Projections, *Health Care Financing Review,* vol. 2, no. 3, (Winter 1981), pp. 97-138.

6. Almost all Medicaid spending goes for provider payments; only about 5 percent goes for program administration. In FY 1979, program administration accounted for $1.1 billion, compared with $20.55 billion for provider payments. Muse and Sawyer, *Medicare and Medicaid Data Book, 1981.*

7. Jane Roberts, "States Respond to Tough Fiscal Challenges," *Intergovernmental Perspectives*, vol. 6, no. 2, Spring 1980.

8. The IHPP survey.

9. Ibid.

10. See Holahan, "1982 Medicaid Program Adjustments."

NOTES TO CHAPTER 2

1. Some of the recent drop may be due to improved reporting from New York, which earlier had overstated recipients. See Medicaid/Medicare Management Institute, *Data on the Medicaid Program,* p. 109, technical note 7.

2. Congressional Budget Office, *Medicaid: Choices for 1982 and Beyond,* June 1981.

3. Robert Gibson, "National Health Care Expenditures, 1979," *Health Care Financing Review,* vol. 2, no. 1 (Summer 1980), pp. 1-36.

4. Medicaid grew from $8.6 to $20.5 billion, Medicare from $9.6 to $29.3 billion, all private medical spending from $63.9 to $124.5 billion, and hospital costs from $102.30 per day to $217.10. Data are from Muse and Sawyer *Medicare and Medicaid Data Book;* Robert M. Gibson and Daniel R. Waldo, "National Health Expenditures, 1980," *Health Care Financing Review,* vol. 3, no. 1, (September 1981), pp. 1-54; and Health Insurance Association of America, Source Book of Health Insurance Data, 1981-1982.

5. Thomas W. Grannemann, "Reforming National Health Programs for the Poor," in M. Pauly, ed., *National Health Insurance* (Washington, D.C.: American Enterprise Institute, 1980), pp. 103-36.

6. One measure of generosity is the spending under Medicaid compared with personal income in a state. In 1977, for instance, the national average was $10.73 per $1,000 of personal income. Spending by states varied widely, however, from $2.73 in Wyoming to $22.68 in New York. Considering only the *state* share and not the federal match, the spread is even larger; New York's $11.31 is twelve times Utah's $0.92 per $1,000 income. Muse and Sawyer, *The Medicare and Medicaid Data Book, 1981.*

7. This does not necessarily mean lowering long-term trends of increased spending. Between 1973 and 1979, the average annual increase in Texas was 17.2 percent, which was above the national average of 15.5 percent.

8. Grannemann, "Reforming National Health Programs for the Poor."

9. Some state officials speak wistfully of the possibility of federal Medicaid expansion to provide similar help in the mental health sphere. Current law allows states at their option to cover ICF services in mental disease institutions only for people age sixty-five or older. Such expansion is extremely unlikely to occur. Not only do the mentally ill seem politically less attractive beneficiaries than the retarded, but also the current federal climate of austerity also militates against any such expansion.

10. Judith Feder and William Scanlon, "Program Transfers in Long Term Care: Strategies to Maintain Service at Minimal State Expense," Urban Institute Working Paper 1466-15, December 1981.

NOTES TO CHAPTER 3

1. See e.g., Bruce Spitz, *State Guide to Medicaid Cost Containment,* (Washinton, D.C.: The Intergovernmental Health Policy Project and the National Governors Association, September 1981); previous Urban Institute work (note 2 to Introduction and Summary); and Jerome Chapman, Toshio Tatara, and Nancy Greenspan, *Federal Regulations, Statutes, and Reporting Requirements as Barriers to Efficient Medicaid Program Operations* (HCFA: Health Care Financing Grants and Contracts Report, Pub. No. 03120, July 1981).

2. For a fuller description of pre-1981 law and practice, see Marilyn Rymer, Gene Oksman, Judith Dernberg, Particia Benner, and David Ellwood, *Final Report: A Comprehensive Review of Medicaid Eligibility* (Cambridge, Mass.: Urban Systems Research & Engineering, October 1977); and Bruce Spitz and John Holahan, *Modifying Medicaid Eligibility and Benefits* (Washington, D.C.: The Urban Institute, June 1977).

3. For a state-by-state listing of optional services covered as of September 1980, see table 4.7 in Muse and Sawyer, *The Medicare and Medicaid Data Book, 1981.*

4. Bruce Stuart, *State Regulation of Health Services Utilization* (Washington, D.C.: The Urban Institute, June 1979).

5. Mary Ann Allard and Gail E. Toft, *Current and Future Development of Intermediate Care Facilities for the Mentally Retarded* (Washington, D.C.: The Intergovernmental Health Policy Project, August 1980).

6. Karen Sheridan, "Analysis of State Medicaid Plan Changes for the Period July 1978 to June 1980," (HCFA internal memo, January 1981).

7. Rate setting is often called "prospective" payment to emphasize the goal of getting hospitals to live within an advance budget. In practice, such regulation often sets rates concurrently or retrospectively, sometimes with adjustments after the end of a fiscal year.

8. See Craig Coelen and Daniel Sullivan, "An Analysis of the Effects of Prospective Reimbursement Programs on Hospital Expenditures," *Health Care Financing Review* vol. 2, no. 3 (Winter 1981), pp. 1-40, and sources cited therein.

9. Ibid.

72   MEDICAID IN THE REAGAN ERA

10. An appeals court ultimately held that a fixed percentage cap might theoretically be permissible but that California's cap had been insufficiently reviewed by
the federal Department of Health, Education and Welfare to have been administratively approvable. *California Hospital Association* v. *Obledo,* 602 F.2nd 1357 (9th
Cir. 1979).

11. Randall R. Bovbjerg, "The Effects of the Courts on Health Care Regulation:
The Case of Hospital Rate Setting," Urban Institute Working Paper No.1393-02,
October 1981.

12. *California Hospital Association* v. *Schweiker (and consolidated cases),* No.
CV 82-0297-CHH (JRx), U.S. District Court, Cent. Dist. of Calif., June 23, 1982.

13. California Assembly Bill No. 799, Section 17, adding Article 2.6 to the Welfare and Institutions Code.

14. There is a chicken-and-egg causation problem here. Medicaid's often strict
fiscal constraints, when coupled with lax monitoring of quality and inadequate enforcement authority, can exacerbate problems by driving out legitimate high-quality
homes while inadvertently allowing good returns to unscrupulous operators.

15. John Holahan, Janet Gornick, and Daniel Nichols, "Physicians' Fees in State
Medicaid Programs," Urban Institute Working Paper 1298-9, (rev). October 1981.

16. The three states averaging higher Medicaid than Medicare fees may or may
not have been in technical violation of the former rule that Medicaid fees not exceed
Medicare fees. There are several explanations for higher Medicaid fees; for a detailed
explanation, see John Holahan, "A Comparison of Medicaid and Medicare Physician
Reimbursement Rates," Urban Institute Working Paper 1306-02-04, March 1982.

17. Gibson, "National Health Care Expenditures, 1979."

18. Philip J. Held, John Holahan, and Cathy Carlson, "The Effect of Medicaid
and Private Fees on Physician Participation in California's Medicaid Program, 1974-
1978," Urban Institute Working Paper 1306-02-01, March 1982. Physician willingness to participate may also be adversely affected by features of a Medicaid program
other than low fees: heavy paperwork, slow payment, intrusive utilization review,
and inability to prescribe drugs or other treatment as desired because of program
restrictions.

19. See, for example, Holahan, Gornick, and Nichols, "Physicians' Fees in State
Medicaid Programs."

20. Harold S. Luft, *Health Maintenance Organizations: Dimensions of Performance* (New York: Wiley, 1981); Harold S. Luft, "How Do Health Maintenance Organization Achieve Their 'Savings'? Rhetoric and Evidence," *New England Journal
of Medicine,* vol. 298, no. 24 (June 15, 1978), pp.1336-43.

21. Margaret Stassen and John Holahan, "Long-Term Care Demonstration Projects: A Review of Recent Evaluations," Urban Institute Working Paper 1227-02,
February 1981.